# Study Guide and Review Manual of

# Human Embryology

## Third Edition

### KEITH L. MOORE

**KEITH L. MOORE, M.Sc., Ph.D., F.I.A.C.**

Professor of Anatomy and Associate Dean, Basic Sciences
University of Toronto, Faculty of Medicine,
Toronto, Ontario, Canada.

Formerly Head of Anatomy in the University of Manitoba and then
Chairman of the Department at the University of Toronto

1988

**W.B. SAUNDERS COMPANY**
Harcourt Brace Jovanovich, Inc.

Philadelphia / London / Toronto / Montreal / Sydney / Tokyo

W. B. Saunders Company
Harcourt Brace Jovanovich, Inc.

The Curtis Center
Independence Square West
Philadelphia, PA   19106

MOORE: STUDY GUIDE & REVIEW MANUAL OF HUMAN EMBRYOLOGY 3/E     ISBN 0-7216-2412-X

Printed in the United States of America

Last digit is the print number 9 8 7 6 5 4 3 2

To our son Warren

in recognition of his success in television

electronics technology

# PREFACE

xxxxxxxxxxxxxxxxxxxxxxxxxxxxxxxxxxxxxxxxxxxxxxxxxxxxxxxxxxxxxxxxxxxxxxxxxxxxxxxxxxxxxx

This Study Guide and Review Manual is designed primarily for use with the author's textbooks: *The Developing Human: Clinically Oriented Embryology* and *Before We Are Born: Basic Embryology and Birth Defects*, published by the W. B. Saunders Company. However, it can be used with similar advantage by students using other textbooks of human embryology.

This book is designed as a *study guide* for beginning students and a *review manual* for advanced students preparing for National Board and other examinations. Because multiple-choice examinations are being used more and more, and are formidable even to the best prepared, commonly used types of these questions have been developed around each topic in embryology. These test questions are intended for those wishing to determine the state of their knowledge and to improve their skills with multiple-choice exams.

With less time available for the formal study of embryology, there is a need for more independent study by students. To learn independently, stated objectives are required. At the beginning of each chapter in this book, there is a *list of objectives* indicating what students should be able to do when they have completed their study of the topics. The self-assessment questions in each chapter provide students with feedback as to their status in achieving the objectives, and afford them the opportunity to correct deficits that may exist in their knowledge. Encouraging students to use this study guide should not be regarded as 'spoon feeding' because only those students who attempt the questions and study the notes and explanations accompanying the answers will be 'nourished'.

The letters I have received from students around the world expressing their appreciation of this *Study Guide and Review Manual of Embryology* stimulated me to update it. I am grateful to many colleagues, especially Dr. J.W.A. Duckworth, Professor Emeritus, University of Toronto, and Dr. T.V.N. Persaud, Professor and Head of Anatomy at the University of Manitoba, for their help and encouragement. I am especially grateful to my wife Marion who typed this camera ready manuscript, and was the copy editor.

*Toronto, Canada*                                        *Keith L. Moore*

## USER'S GUIDE

xxxxxxxxxxxxxxxxxxxxxxxxxxxxxxxxxxxxxxxxxxxxxxxxxxxxxxxxxxxxxxxxxxxxxxxxxxxx

This study guide is designed to help you study and later review human embryology by providing learning objectives and various types of multiple-choice questions based on these objectives. The guide is not intended as a substitute for careful study of your textbook and lecture notes, but is designed to enable you to detect areas of weakness and afford you the opportunity to correct deficits in your knowledge.

Although the answers to the questions are explained and relevant notes are given, you should consult your textbook for a comprehensive review of difficult concepts and processes. Through discussion of weak areas with your colleagues and instructors, you can test your ability to do the things listed as learning objectives. To use this guide most effectively, the following steps are suggested:

1.  Read the objectives listed at the beginning of the chapter you plan to study.

2.  Carefully study the appropriate chapter in your textbook, focusing on the topics included in the objectives.

3.  Attempt the series of questions: five-choice completion, multi-completion and five-choice association. All questions are designed to be answered at the rate of about one per minute. As you complete each set of questions, check your answers. If any of your answers are wrong, read the notes and explanations and study the appropriate material and illustrations in your textbook before proceeding to the next set of questions.

4.  If you get 80 per cent or more of the questions correct on the first trial, or during a subsequent review, you have performed very well and should have no difficulty answering similar questions based on the objectives given in this guide.

# C O N T E N T S

xxxxxxxxxxxxxxxxxxxxxxxxxxxxxxxxxxxxxxxxxxxxxxxxxxxxxxxxxxxxxxxxxxxxxxxxxxxx

Contents Continued.

Contents Continued.

# INTRODUCTION TO EMBRYOLOGY

Terms and Concepts

## O B J E C T I V E S

BE ABLE TO:

---

o  Define the term development and name the developmental
   periods*.
o  Differentiate between the terms conceptus and abortus.
o  Explain why embryology forms a basis for medical and dental
   practice.
o  Differentiate between the terms embryology and teratology.
o  Use the various terms of position and direction, and to illustrate the various planes of the body.
o  Explain the difference in meaning between the following terms:
   embryo and fetus; conception and conceptus; embryology and developmental anatomy; and embryology and teratology.

---

## F I V E - C H O I C E  C O M P L E T I O N  Q U E S T I O N S

DIRECTIONS:  Each of the following statements or questions is followed by five
suggested responses or completions.  SELECT THE ONE BEST ANSWER in each case and
then circle the appropriate letter at the right of each question.

1.  The term conceptus includes all structures which develop from the

    A.  chorion              D.  trophoblast
    B.  embryoblast          E.  inner cell mass
    C.  zygote                                            A B C D E

---

*Make no attempt to memorize the Timetables of Human Prenatal Development.  Use
them as you would a calendar to indicate important events.

## SELECT THE ONE BEST ANSWER

2. Select the best term for describing the foot with reference to the leg.

   A. Distal
   B. Ventral
   C. Posterior
   D. Inferior
   E. Proximal                                              A B C D E

3. A section through an embryo dividing it into ventral and dorsal parts is a _____ section.

   A. cross           D. oblique
   B. sagittal        E. median
   C. frontal                                               A B C D E

4. In the adult the neck is superior to the thorax. The corresponding term for a fetus is

   A. dorsal
   B. inferior
   C. caudal
   D. ventral
   E. cranial                                               A B C D E

5. The plane dividing a fetus into right and left halves is called the _____ plane.

   A. sagittal
   B. median
   C. coronal
   D. transverse
   E. frontal                                               A B C D E

6. Which of the following embryological terms means 'toward the nose'?

   A. Dorsad          D. Rostral
   B. Cephalic        E. Caudal
   C. Cranial                                               A B C D E

7. Each of the following terms of comparison is used correctly EXCEPT:

   A. The wrist is distal to the forearm.
   B. The brain is located cranial to the spinal cord.
   C. The upper limb arises caudal to the heart.
   D. The knee is proximal to the ankle.
   E. The tail of the embryo is caudal to the abdomen.      A B C D E

======================== ANSWERS, NOTES, AND EXPLANATIONS =========================

1. C  The term conceptus is used when referring to the embryo (or fetus) and its membranes, i.e., the total products of conception which develop from the zygote. The conceptus (embryo and its membranes) expelled or removed during an abortion is called an abortus.

2. A  The foot is at the distal end of the leg. The term distal is commonly used in descriptions of a limb instead of the term inferior.

3. C  A vertical section through the frontal (coronal) plane is known as a frontal (coronal) section. This is one of the major planes of the body.

4. E  The neck of a fetus is cranial (cephalic) to the thorax; i.e., it is closer to the head. Cranial means 'toward the cranium' and cephalic indicates 'toward the brain'.

5. B  The median plane is a vertical plane passing through the center of the body, dividing it into right and left halves. The median plane passes longitudinally through the embryo and intersects the surface of the front and back of the body at what are called the anteromedian and posteromedian lines.

6. D  The term rostral is used to indicate the relationship of structures to the nose (L. rostrum, a beak). For example, the upper lip develops rostral to the eye.

7. C  The upper limb arises slightly cranial to the heart. The Latin term cauda means the tail.


## F I V E - C H O I C E   A S S O C I A T I O N   Q U E S T I O N S

DIRECTIONS: Each group of questions below consists of a numbered list of descriptive words or phrases accompanied by a diagram with certain parts indicated by letters, or by a list of lettered headings. For each numbered word or phrase, SELECT THE LETTERED PART OR HEADING that matches it correctly. Then insert the letter in the space to the right of the appropriate number. Sometimes more than one numbered word or phrase may be correctly matched to the same lettered part or heading.

A. Median          C. Coronal          E. Rostral
B. Dorsal          D. Caudal

1. ____ Posterior              4. ____ Midsagittal
2. ____ Toward the nose        5. ____ Toward the tail
3. ____ Frontal                6. ____ Lying in the middle

## ASSOCIATION QUESTIONS

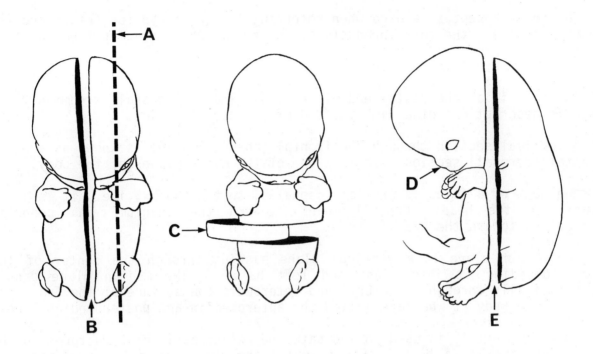

7. _____ Transverse plane
8. _____ Rostral
9. _____ Median plane

10. _____ Frontal plane
11. _____ Sagittal plane
12. _____ Coronal plane


======================= ANSWERS, NOTES, AND EXPLANATIONS =========================


1.   B  Dorsal refers to structures near the back.  In the adult, 'dorsal' is equivalent to 'posterior'.  The term dorsal is commonly used in descriptions of embryos and in some descriptions of adults, e.g., we refer to the dorsum or dorsal part of the foot and hand.

2.   E  Structures that are near the nose are rostral, e.g., a structure such as a nerve grows rostrally (toward the nose) or in a rostral direction.

3.   C  The term 'coronal' is often used synonymously with 'frontal'.  Coronal refers to the fact that a coronal plane passes through the coronal suture of the skull.

4

4.  A  A midsagittal section passes through the median plane. Thus the terms midsagittal and median are used synonymously in reference to sections cut in the median plane, but the term median is preferable.

5.  D  'Caudal' is used in the description of structures that are near the tail or rump of the embryo. Embryos have tails until the early part of the eighth week. In descriptions of adult anatomy, the term 'inferior' is used to indicate structures that are lower in the body, e.g., the large intestine is inferior to the stomach.

6.  A  'Median' means lying in the median plane or midline, and the term 'medial' is used to indicate a structure nearer the median plane, e.g., the eye is medial to the auricle or external ear.

7.  C  The transverse plane is any plane that is at right angles to both the median and frontal planes. Although the term transverse is often used synonymously with horizontal, you must understand that transverse implies that it is through the longitudinal axis of a structure. In the anatomical position, a transverse section through the hand is horizontal, but a transverse section through the foot in the anatomical position is coronal. Transverse sections are used very commonly in embryology, e.g., serial transverse sections of chick and pig embryos are often studied in the laboratory.

8.  D  The term rostral (toward the nose) is used to indicate the relationship of a structure to the nose, e.g., the eyes are rostral to the ears.

9.  B  The median plane is a vertical plane passing through the center of the body, dividing it into right and left halves. Median sections of embryos show the relationship of thoracic and abdominal structures to each other.

10. E  A frontal plane is any vertical plane that intersects the median plane at a right angle. This kind of section is helpful in studying paired structures (e.g., the kidneys), and those that run longitudinally (e.g., the esophagus).

11. A  A sagittal plane is any vertical plane passing through the body parallel to the median plane. A median section passes through the median plane. These sections are often used to show the course of structures that run through various regions of the body, e.g., the esophagus runs through the neck and thorax.

12. E  A frontal plane is often called a coronal plane because a frontal plane passes through the coronal suture of the skull. It divides the body into ventral and dorsal parts. Sections through the frontal plane are commonly used in studying embryos.

NOTES:

# THE BEGINNING OF HUMAN DEVELOPMENT

The First Week

## O B J E C T I V E S

BE ABLE TO:

___

o  Describe spermatogenesis and oogenesis with special emphasis on the chromosomal changes occurring during maturation of the germ cells.

o  Compare the sperm and the ovum with reference to: size; chromosome constitution; time of formation; transport; and viability.

o  Define the term nondisjunction and explain how this abnormal process leads to monosomy and trisomy. Describe the most common malformation syndrome resulting from nondisjunction.

o  Discuss the ovarian cycle (follicle development, ovulation, and corpus luteum formation) and the menstrual cycle, explaining how ovarian cyclic activity is intimately linked with cyclic changes in the endometrium.

o  Discuss capacitation and the acrosome reaction of the sperm.

o  Construct and label simple diagrams illustrating fertilization. List the results of fertilization.

o  Discuss cleavage of the zygote and implantation of the blastocyst, using labelled sketches. Define: blastocyst, zona pellucida, trophoblast, inner cell mass, blastocyst cavity, embryonic pole, embryoblast, blastocyst cavity, and hypoblast.

___

## F I V E - C H O I C E   C O M P L E T I O N   Q U E S T I O N S

DIRECTIONS: Each of the following statements or questions is followed by five suggested responses or completions. SELECT THE ONE BEST ANSWER in each case and then circle the appropriate letter at the right of each question.

1.  Prior to ejaculation, sperms are stored chiefly in the

   A.  seminal vesicles
   B.  efferent ductules
   C.  ejaculatory ducts
   D.  epididymis
   E.  rete testis

   A B C D E

SELECT THE ONE BEST ANSWER

2.  Which of the following types of germ cell does not undergo cell division?

    A.  Spermatogonia          D.  Secondary spermatocytes
    B.  Primary oocytes         E.  Oogonia
    C.  Spermatids                                              A B C D E

3.  Which of the following chromosome constitutions in a sperm normally results in a male, if it fertilizes an ovum?

    A.  22, 0          D.  23, X
    B.  22, X          E.  23, Y
    C.  22, Y                                                   A B C D E

4.  Oogonia are homologous to spermatogonia.  They divide by mitosis during

    A.  all postnatal periods    D.  the reproductive period
    B.  early fetal life          E.  none of the above
    C.  puberty                                                A B C D E

5.  The normal chromosome number of a human spermatid is

    A.  23 autosomes plus two different sex chromosomes
    B.  22 autosomes plus an X and a Y chromosome
    C.  23 autosomes plus two identical sex chromosomes
    D.  22 autosomes plus an X or a Y chromosome
    E.  46, XY                                                 A B C D E

6.  Morphologically abnormal sperms may cause

    A.  monosomy               D.  abnormal embryos
    B.  congenital malformations E.  infertility
    C.  trisomy                                                A B C D E

7.  Which of the following layers of the embryo is recognizable at the end of the first week of development?

    A.  Hypoblast              D.  Epiblast
    B.  Mesoderm               E.  Somatopleure
    C.  Ectoderm                                               A B C D E

8.  The secondary oocyte completes the second meiotic division

    A.  before ovulation       D.  before birth
    B.  during ovulation       E.  at puberty
    C.  at fertilization                                       A B C D E

SELECT THE ONE BEST ANSWER

9.  The sperm penetrates the zona pellucida, digesting a path by
    the action of enzymes released from the ____ of the sperm.

    A.  middle piece          D.  main piece
    B.  acrosome              E.  head
    C.  neck                                      A B C D E

10. How many sperms would likely be deposited by a normal young
    adult male in the vagina during intercourse?

    A.  300 thousand
    B.  3 million
    C.  30 million
    D.  300 million
    E.  3 billion                                 A B C D E


===================== ANSWERS, NOTES, AND EXPLANATIONS ==========================


1.  D  Sperms are stored and undergo further maturation in the epididymis.  They
    are not stored in the seminal vesicles as was believed for many years.
    During ejaculation the sperms are forced through the ductus deferens into the
    urethra from which they are expelled with the secretions of the accessory
    glands (e.g., the prostate) as semen.  If not ejaculated, the sperms degener-
    ate and are absorbed within the epididymis.

2.  C  Spermatids do not divide.  They are gradually transformed during spermio-
    genesis into mature sperms.  Spermatogonia and oogonia undergo mitosis.
    Primary spermatocytes and oocytes undergo the first meiotic division.

3.  E  Fertilization of an ovum by a Y sperm (i.e., 23, Y) produces a 46, XY
    zygote which normally develops into a male.  The number 46 designates the
    total number of chromosomes, including the two sex chromosomes (XY).  This is
    the accepted way of indicating the chromosome composition of cells.  The sex
    of the embryo depends upon whether an X or a Y sperm fertilizes the ovum.
    The mother can contribute only an X chromosome and so cannot determine the
    embryo's sex.

4.  B  Oogonia proliferate during the early fetal period and, unlike spermato-
    gonia, do not begin to increase at puberty.  All oogonia become primary
    oocytes before birth.  Many of the two million or so oocytes present in both
    ovaries at birth degenerate before puberty, leaving not more than 30,000 to
    undergo further development after puberty.

5.  D  Spermatids are haploid cells (23 chromosomes) which have 22 autosomes plus
    a Y or an X chromosome, i.e., one or the other but not both.  Thus, the
    haploid number in man is 23.  If two members of a chromosome pair fail to

separate (nondisjunction), abnormal spermatids can have 22 autosomes and two sex chromosomes, or no sex chromosome.

6. E  It is generally believed that structurally abnormal sperms do not fertilize ova because of their lack of normal motility and fertilizing power. Examination of semen is important in the study of fertility. The number, motility, and abnormalities in size and shape of sperms are important in assessing sterility in males. If 20 per cent or more sperms are morphologically abnormal, fertility is usually impaired.

7. A  The bilaminar embryonic disc forms early in the second week. At the end of the first week, the hypoblast (primitive endoderm) begins to form on the ventral surface of the inner cell mass. The epiblast, which gives rise to the embryonic ectoderm and mesoderm, is not recognizable until the beginning of the second week, when the amniotic cavity forms.

8. C  When a sperm contacts the cell membrane of a secondary oocyte, the oocyte completes the second maturation or meiotic division and becomes a mature ovum or oocyte. The second polar body, a nonfunctional cell, is formed during this division. If fertilization does not occur, the secondary oocyte does not complete this division; it degenerates within 24 hours after ovulation.

9. B  It is believed that the sperm digests a path for itself through the corona radiata by the action of an enzyme, hyaluronidase, released from the sperm's acrosome through perforations that develop in it during the acrosome reaction. Movements of the tail of the sperm may also be involved in this process.

10. D  At least 300 million sperms are deposited in the vagina at intercourse. Usually 200 - 600 million sperms are in the ejaculate, but only a few hundred sperms are believed to reach the fertilization site. If less than 50 million sperms are present in a semen sample, the male from whom the sample was taken may be infertile.


M U L T I - C O M P L E T I O N   Q U E S T I O N S


DIRECTIONS:  In each of the following questions or incomplete statements ONE OR MORE of the completions is correct. At the lower right of each question, circle A if 1, 2, and 3 are correct; B if 1 and 3 are correct; C if 2 and 4 are correct; D if only 4 is correct; and E if all are correct.


1. With the light microscope, the zona pellucida appears as a translucent membrane surrounding the

    1. primary oocyte
    2. morula
    3. zygote
    4. early blastocyst                                    A B C D E

| A | B | C | D | E |
|---|---|---|---|---|
| 1,2,3 | 1,3 | 2,4 | only 4 | all correct |

2. Parts of the four-day blastocyst include the

    1. trophoblast
    2. zona pellucida
    3. inner cell mass
    4. syncytiotrophoblast                           A B C D E

3. The human morula forms about three days after fertilization and usually

    1. contains a single fluid-filled cavity
    2. consists of 16 or so blastomeres
    3. remains in the uterine tube for two days
    4. enters the uterus three days after fertilization     A B C D E
                                 *it forms*

4. Development of an ovarian follicle is characterized by

    1. growth and differentiation of the primary oocyte
    2. proliferation of follicular cells surrounding the oocyte
    3. development of the theca folliculi around the follicle
    4. formation of the membranous zona pellucida     A B C D E

5. As implantation of the blastocyst occurs, the trophoblast differentiates into the

    1. cytotrophoblast            3. syncytiotrophoblast
    2. embryoblast               4. embryotroph     A B C D E

6. Results of fertilization include:

    1. restoration of the diploid number
    2. dispersion of the corona radiata
    3. determination of the embryo's sex
    4. maturation of the sperm or gamete     A B C D E

7. The seven-day blastocyst

    1. has a double layer of trophoblast at the embryonic pole
    2. has an amniotic cavity
    3. is attached to the endometrial epithelium
    4. is surrounded by a degenerating zona pellucida     A B C D E

8. The first week of human development is characterized by formation of the

    1. inner cell mass            3. trophoblast
    2. hypoblast               4. blastocyst     A B C D E

| A | B | C | D | E |
|---|---|---|---|---|
| 1,2,3 | 1,3, | 2,4 | only 4 | all correct |

9.  Correct statements about the morula include:

    1.  All of its blastomeres have a similar appearance.
    2.  The zona pellucida surrounding it is partially deficient.
    3.  It has a group of centrally located cells (inner cell mass).
    4.  It enters the uterus about three days after it forms.        A B C D E

10. Correct statements about cleavage of the zygote include:

    1.  consists of a series of rapid meiotic divisions
    2.  results in the formation of increasingly smaller cells
    3.  begins when the pronuclei contact each other
    4.  occurs as the zygote passes down the uterine tube        A B C D E

11. Events occurring when a sperm contacts the cell membrane of an oocyte include:

    1.  The oocyte completes the second meiotic division.
    2.  The sperm undergoes capacitation.
    3.  Changes occur in the zona pellucida preventing penetration by other sperms.
    4.  The tail of the sperm undergoes degeneration.        A B C D E

12. Before a sperm is capable of fertilizing an ovum, it must

    1.  undergo a physiological change called capacitation
    2.  completely penetrate the corona radiata and the zona pellucida
    3.  undergo a structural change called the acrosome reaction
    4.  complete the second meiotic division and become a mature sperm        A B C D E


======================= ANSWERS, NOTES, AND EXPLANATIONS =========================


1.  E  All are correct.  As the primary oocyte grows, the zona pellucida develops around it, separating it from the follicular cells of the growing ovarian follicle.  This amorphous extracellular layer remains around the secondary oocyte during ovulation and, if the ovum is fertilized, it surrounds the zygote and morula.  During cleavage the zona pellucida keeps the blastomeres together and prevents their adherence to the epithelium of the uterine tube. The zona pellucida also surrounds the early blastocyst, but as this structure expands the zona pellucida degenerates and disappears by the fifth day after fertilization.

2.  B  1 and 3 are correct.  The zona pellucida surrounds the blastocyst, but is

not part of it. The syncytiotrophoblast does not form until implantation begins at the end of the first week. Usually by the seventh day, the syncytiotrophoblast has penetrated the endometrial epithelium. The inner cell mass is the part of the blastocyst which gives rise to the embryo. The trophoblast later becomes part of the chorion which gives rise to the embryonic part of the placenta.

3.  C  2 and 4 are correct.  The morula does not contain a cavity and it does not remain in the uterine tube for two days.  As soon as a cavity forms, the developing human is referred to as a blastocyst.  The morula enters the uterus shortly after it forms, usually about three days after fertilization. It develops into a blastocyst about a day later.

4.  E  All are correct.  As the ovarian follicle develops, the primary oocyte enlarges and the follicular cells around it proliferate.  The amorphous extra-cellular layer, known as the zona pellucida, develops between the primary oocyte and the follicular cells.  The connective tissue surrounding the follicle differentiates into the theca folliculi.

5.  B  1 and 3 are correct.  The trophoblast differentiates into two layers: cytotrophoblast and syncytiotrophoblast.  It does not differentiate into the inner cell mass (embryoblast) or the embryotroph.  Embryotroph is a nutrient fluid composed of maternal blood, glandular secretions, and the remains of degenerated cells.

6.  B  1 and 3 are correct.  The other main result of fertilization is initiation of cleavage (mitotic division) of the zygote.  Fertilization is also the physical basis for biparental inheritance and the method for bringing about variation of the human species.  The initiation of fertilization also prevents other sperms from penetrating the ovum; stimulates the secondary oocyte to complete the second meiotic division; and leads to extrusion of the second polar body, a nonfunctional cell that soon degenerates.

7.  B  1 and 3 are correct.  The seven-day blastocyst has a double layer of trophoblast, cytotrophoblast and syncytiotrophoblast, at the site of attachment, almost always at the embryonic pole (i.e., adjacent to the inner cell mass).  The blastocyst is superficially attached to the endometrial epithelium, but the amniotic cavity is not recognizable until the eighth day. The zona pellucida usually disappears by the fifth day after fertilization.

8.  E  All are correct.  As soon as a cavity forms in the morula, it is referred to as a blastocyst which consists of: (1) an inner cell mass or embryoblast which gives rise to the embryo; (2) a blastocyst cavity; and (3) an outer layer of cells or the trophoblast.  The hypoblast (primitive endoderm) begins to form on the ventral surface of the inner cell mass at the end of the first week.  Most of the cells in this layer are probably displaced to extra-embryonic regions, e.g., into the wall of the yolk sac.

9.  B  1 and 3 are true.  Although all cells of the morula appear similar, the central cells (inner cell mass) will give rise to the embryo.  The future trophoblast will form from the outer cell layer.  The zona pellucida does not begin to degenerate until the fourth or fifth day after fertilization.  As the morula forms, it enters the uterus (about day 3).

10. C **2 and 4 are true.** Cleavage consists of a rapid series of mitotic (not meiotic) cell divisions. The zygote does not undergo meiosis or reduction divisions. Cleavage produces a progressively larger number of increasingly smaller cells, called blastomeres. Division of the zygote does not begin until after the male and female pronuclei have fused to form the nucleus of the zygote. Cleavage of the zygote occurs as it passes down the uterine tube to the uterus; the journey takes about three days.

11. B **1 and 3 are correct.** The secondary oocyte reacts to sperm contact in two ways: (1) changes occur in the zona pellucida and in the oocyte's cell membrane which inhibit the entry of more sperms, and (2) the secondary oocyte completes the second meiotic division and becomes a mature ovum. The head and tail of the sperm enter the ovum's cytoplasm, but the cell membrane of the sperm stays outside. The tail soon degenerates, apparently becoming absorbed by the cytoplasm of the ovum. Freshly ejaculated sperms are incapable of fertilizing ova; they must undergo capacitation. This physiological process is believed to take up to eight hours and seems to depend upon intimate contact between the sperms and the endometrial epithelium.

12. A **1, 2, and 3 are correct.** To be capable of fertilizing an ovum, a sperm must undergo capacitation and later the acrosome reaction. The enzyme hyaluronidase released from the acrosome disperses the cells of the corona radiata. There is evidence that an enzyme secreted by the tubal mucosa may also be required for dispersal of the corona radiata. Hyaluronidase and another enzyme from the acrosome digest a path through the zona pellucida for the sperm to follow. Once through the zona pellucida, the sperm contacts the oocyte and the actual fertilization process begins. Several sperms may penetrate the corona radiata and begin to pass through the zona pellucida, but normally only one sperm penetrates the cell membrane of the oocyte and enters its cytoplasm. Neither spermatids nor sperms undergo cell division. Spermatids are transformed into mature sperms during the stage of spermatogenesis called spermiogenesis.

## F I V E - C H O I C E   A S S O C I A T I O N   Q U E S T I O N S

DIRECTIONS: Each group of questions below consists of a numbered list of descriptive words or phrases accompanied by a diagram with certain parts indicated by letters, or by a list of lettered headings. For each numbered word or phrase, SELECT THE LETTERED PART OR HEADING that matches it correctly. Then insert the letter in the space to the right of the appropriate number. Sometimes more than one numbered word or phrase may be correctly matched to the same lettered part or heading.

A.  Polar bodies      B.  Capacitation      C.  Acrosome
D.  Zona pellucida    E.  Pronuclei

1. _____ Haploid nuclei which fuse to form a zygote
2. _____ Changes occur in it that inhibit entry of sperms
3. _____ Contains enzymes that digest a path for the sperm
4. _____ Nonfunctional cells produced during oogenesis

## ASSOCIATION QUESTIONS

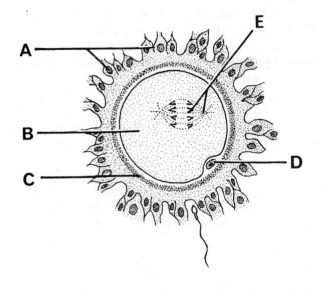

5. _____ Polar body
6. _____ Zona pellucida
7. _____ Diploid cells
8. _____ Meiotic spindle
9. _____ Corona radiata
10. _____ Haploid cell

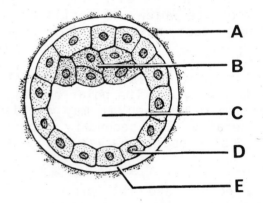

11. _____ Embryoblast
12. _____ Gives rise to part of the placenta
13. _____ Gives rise to the embryo
14. _____ Gives rise to the hypoblast
15. _____ Degenerates and disappears
16. _____ Blastocyst cavity

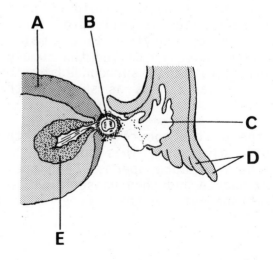

17. _____ Once filled the follicular antrum
18. _____ Develops under LH influence
19. _____ Produces progesterone
20. _____ Expelled with the follicular fluid
21. _____ Fimbriae
22. _____ Derived from a primary oocyte

======================== ANSWERS, NOTES, AND EXPLANATIONS =========================

1.    E   The male and female pronuclei are the haploid nuclei of the sperm and the ovum, respectively.  They fuse during fertilization to form the diploid nucleus of a zygote.  The nucleus occupies most of the head of the sperm and after it enters the ovum, it swells to form the male pronucleus.  The pronuclei are of approximately equal size and show similar features.

2.    D   The zona pellucida undergoes changes, called the zona reaction, when a sperm contacts the cell membrane of a secondary oocyte.  These changes, caused by the release of substances from the oocyte, prevent other sperms from passing through the zona pellucida and entering the oocyte.

3.    C   The acrosome is a cap-like structure that invests the anterior half of the head of the sperm.  It contains enzymes which pass through perforations in its wall and digest a path for the sperm to follow through the zona pellucida to contact the oocyte.

4.    A   The polar bodies are small haploid cells that are produced during the first and second meiotic divisions.  The polar bodies have the same number of chromosomes as the secondary and mature oocytes, but they receive very little cytoplasm.  Most cytoplasm goes to the mature oocyte which, if fertilized, contributes to the zygote.  The sperm probably does not contribute any cytoplasm to the zygote.

5.    D   The first polar body forms during the first meiotic division.  Note that it is inside the zona pellucida with the secondary oocyte.  The polar body is a haploid cell and receives very little cytoplasm.  Although it may divide into two polar bodies, all these cells degenerate.  The secondary oocyte receives the same number of chromosomes as the polar body; however, it gets almost all the cytoplasm.

6.    C   The zona pellucida surrounds the secondary oocyte and the polar body.  This membrane is surrounded by a layer of follicular cells called the corona radiata.  The zona pellucida appears homogeneous in the fresh condition, but under the EM it has a granular appearance and shows some concentric layering.

7.    A   The follicular cells of the corona radiata are the only diploid cells in the diagram.  During follicular development, the follicular cells proliferate by mitosis and form a stratified epithelium around the oocyte.  In the mature follicle, the oocyte lies in a mound of follicular cells called the cumulus oophorus.  When the oocyte is expelled at ovulation, it is surrounded by the zona pellucida and one or more layers of follicular cells, as shown in the diagram.

8.    E   Contact of a sperm with the cell membrane of the oocyte stimulates the secondary oocyte to complete its second meiotic division.  This contact also brings about the zona reaction preventing entry of more sperms.  The sperm penetrates the cell membrane of the secondary oocyte and then passes into the cytoplasm of the oocyte, leaving its cell membrane outside the oocyte.

9.  A  As previously described, the corona radiata consists of one or more layers of follicular cells that surround the zona pellucida, the polar body, and the secondary oocyte. The corona radiata is dispersed during fertilization by enzymes released from the acrosomes of the sperms surrounding the ovum.

10. D  The first polar body is a haploid cell formed during the first meiotic division of the oocyte. The sperm is also a haploid cell. The sex chromosomal content of the sperm determines the sex of the zygote. If a sperm with an X chromosome fertilizes an ovum, a zygote forms which normally develops into a female. If a sperm with a Y chromosome fertilizes an ovum, a zygote forms which normally develops into a male. As there are equal numbers of X and Y sperms, the chances of a male or female zygote resulting from fertilization are equal. Despite this, more males than females are born.

11. B  The embryoblast or inner cell mass is recognizable about four days after fertilization. It is derived from the central cells of the morula. The embryoblast gives rise to the embryo.

12. D  The outer cell layer of the blastocyst (trophoblast) gives rise to the embryonic part of the placenta; the other part is derived from the endometrium. When the trophoblast becomes lined by extraembryonic somatic mesoderm, the combined layers are called the chorion. The trophoblast forms no part of the embryo.

13. B  The embryoblast or inner cell mass gives rise to the embryo. The first sign of differentiation of the inner cell mass is the appearance of the hypoblast on its ventral surface. The inner cell mass later gives rise to two more germ layers. The three germ layers give rise to all the tissues and organs of the embryo.

14. B  At the end of the first week, differentiation of the inner cell mass gives rise to the hypoblast. It appears as a flattened layer on the ventral surface of the inner cell mass. Later it will form the roof of the yolk sac and be incorporated into the embryo as the lining of the primitive gut.

15. A  The zona pellucida begins to degenerate about four days after fertilization as the blastocyst begins to expand rapidly. The zona pellucida disappears on the fourth or fifth day. Implantation begins on the sixth day.

16. C  The blastocyst cavity forms as fluid passes into the morula from the uterus and accumulates. The spaces around the central cells of the morula coalesce to form the blastocyst cavity, converting the morula into a blastocyst. The uterine fluid in the blastocyst cavity bathes the ventral surface of the inner cell mass, and probably supplies nutrients to the embryonic cells.

17. C  Follicular fluid fills the antra of growing and mature ovarian follicles. When the stigma ruptures at ovulation, the oocyte is expelled with the fluid from the follicle and the ovary in a few seconds. Expulsion of the ovum and fluid is the result of intrafollicular pressure and possibly from ovarian smooth muscle contraction.

18. E The corpus luteum develops under the influence of LH (luteinizing hormone). It produces progesterone and some estrogen. These hormones act on the endometrium bringing about the secretory phase and preparing the endometrium for implantation of a blastocyst. If the ovum is fertilized, the corpus luteum enlarges into a corpus luteum of pregnancy and increases its hormone production. If the ovum is not fertilized, the corpus luteum begins to degenerate about nine days after ovulation and is called a corpus luteum of menstruation.

19. E The corpus luteum usually produces progesterone for about nine days. However if the ovum is fertilized, it produces progesterone until about the end of the fourth month of pregnancy. If you chose "A" for the answer, you are partly right because the ovary produces progesterone. "E" is a better answer because it is more specific.

20. B The secondary oocyte is expelled with follicular fluid at ovulation. Ovulation is under FSH and LH influence and occurs through the ruptured stigma. The oocyte quickly leaves the peritoneal cavity and enters the infundibulum (L. funnel) of the uterine tube.

21. D The fimbriae of the uterine tube embrace the ovary at ovulation. The sweeping motion of the fimbriae and the motion of the cilia on their epithelial lining cells carry the oocyte into the uterine tube.

22. B The secondary oocyte is derived from a primary oocyte following the first meiotic division. This division produces two haploid cells, the secondary oocyte and the first polar body. By the time of ovulation, the secondary oocyte has begun the second meiotic division, but progresses only to the metaphase stage where division is arrested. If the oocyte is fertilized it will complete the division, forming a mature ovum.

---

NOTES:

# FORMATION OF THE BILAMINAR EMBRYO

The Second Week

## O B J E C T I V E S

BE ABLE TO:

---

o   Describe the implantation of a blastocyst, using simple labelled diagrams.

o   Discuss the proliferation and differentiation of the trophoblast; formation of lacunar networks; and the establishment of the primitive uteroplacental circulation.

o   Trace the development of the amniotic cavity, the bilaminar embryonic disc, the yolk sac, the extraembryonic mesoderm, the extraembryonic coelom, and the connecting stalk.

o   Write brief notes on the following: prochordal plate, embryotroph, chorion, primary chorionic villi, chorionic sac, decidual reaction, and ectopic pregnancies.

---

## F I V E - C H O I C E   C O M P L E T I O N   Q U E S T I O N S

DIRECTIONS: Each of the following statements or questions is followed by five suggested responses or completions. SELECT THE ONE BEST ANSWER in each case and then circle the appropriate letter at the right of each question.

1.   The eight-day blastocyst

A.   has a single layer of trophoblast at the embryonic pole
B.   has lacunae in the syncytiotrophoblast
C.   is partially implanted in the endometrium
D.   is covered by the uterine epithelium
E.   has a primitive yolk sac                              A B C D E

2.   The syncytiotrophoblast

A.   surrounds the 8-day blastocyst
B.   has well defined cell boundaries
C.   shows little invasive activity
D.   is derived from the cytotrophoblast
E.   is nonfunctional                                       A B C D E

## SELECT THE ONE BEST ANSWER

3.  The amniotic cavity develops

    A.  initially on the tenth day
    B.  within the  inner cell mass
    C.  between the inner cell mass and the trophoblast
    D.  in the extraembryonic mesoderm
    E.  during the first week                                           A B C D E

4.  Which statement about the 14-day blastocyst is <u>FALSE</u>?

    A.  Primary chorionic villi are absent.
    B.  Extraembryonic coelom surrounds the yolk sac.
    C.  The primitive uteroplacental circulation is established.
    D.  The extraembryonic mesoderm is split into two layers.
    E.  It is completely implanted in the endometrium.                  A B C D E

5.  In the 10- to 12-day blastocyst,

    A.  the conceptus lies deep to the endometrial epithelium
    B.  the defect in the endometrial epithelium is indicated
        by a closing plug.
    C.  the implanted blastocyst produces a minute elevation on
        the endometrial surface.
    D.  maternal blood begins to flow slowly through the lacunar
        networks
    E.  all of the above are correct                                    A B C D E

6.  The wall of the chorionic sac is composed of

    A.  cytotrophoblast and syncytiotrophoblast
    B.  two layers of trophoblast lined by extraembryonic
        somatic mesoderm
    C.  trophoblast and the exocoelomic membrane
    D.  extraembryonic splanchnic mesoderm and both layers
        of trophoblast
    E.  none of the above is correct                                    A B C D E

7.  During the second week, lacunar networks develop within the

    A.  extraembryonic mesoderm
    B.  inner cell mass
    C.  syncytiotrophoblast
    D.  endometrium
    E.  embryoblast                                                     A B C D E

8.  Ectopic implantations occur most commonly in the

    A.  ovary                      D.  cervix
    B.  abdomen                    E.  peritoneal cavity
    C.  uterine tube                                                    A B C D E

SELECT THE ONE BEST ANSWER

9.  Each of the following is directly involved with early implan-
    tation EXCEPT:

    A.  decidual reaction          D.  invasion
    B.  progesterone               E.  endometrial
    C.  stratum spongiosum             epithelium          A  B  C  D  E


10. The amniotic cavity appears on the eighth day as a slit-like
    space between the trophoblast and the

    A.  extraembryonic mesoderm    D.  connecting stalk
    B.  inner cell mass            E.  chorion
    C.  exocoelomic membrane                           A  B  C  D  E


======================== ANSWERS, NOTES, AND EXPLANATIONS ========================

1.  C  The 8-day blastocyst is partially implanted in the endometrium.  The
    trophoblast at the pole opposite the embryo (abembryonic pole) remains un-
    differentiated, consisting of a thin layer of flattened cytotrophoblastic
    cells.  The trophoblast consists of two layers only where it is in contact
    with the endometrium (usually adjacent to the inner cell mass).  The
    primitive yolk sac is not usually present at eight days, but the amniotic
    cavity is represented by a small slit-like space.

2.  D  The syncytiotrophoblast is derived from the cytotrophoblast.  The cyto-
    trophoblast is mitotically active and forms new cells which fuse with and
    become part of the increasing mass of syncytiotrophoblast.  The syncytiotro-
    phoblast does not enclose the 8-day blastocyst on all sides.  It forms a
    multinucleated protoplasmic mass at the embryonic pole.  The syncytiotropho-
    blast does not have well-defined cell boundaries.  Invasiveness is one of the
    spectacular properties of the syncytiotrophoblast.  The penetration and
    subsequent erosion of the endometrium by the syncytiotrophoblast results from
    proteolytic enzymes produced by the syncytiotrophoblast.

3.  C  The amniotic cavity appears on the eighth day after fertilization between
    the inner cell mass and the invading syncytiotrophoblast.  It does not
    develop in the inner cell mass or in the extraembryonic mesoderm.  The amnion
    forms from cells derived from the cytotrophoblast.

4.  A  Primary chorionic villi are characteristic features of the 14-day
    blastocyst.  All the other statements about the blastocyst at the end of the
    second week are true.

5.  E  These statements about the 10- to 12-day blastocyst are all true.  The
    important statement is D because the presence of maternal blood establishes
    an abundant source of nutrition for the conceptus.

6.  B  The wall of the chorionic sac is composed of the chorion which is formed by the combination of extraembryonic somatic mesoderm and the two layers of trophoblast (cytotrophoblast and syncytiotrophoblast).  The chorionic sac contains the embryo which is attached to its wall by the connecting stalk.

7.  C  Lacunar networks develop in the syncytiotrophoblast by coalescence of lacunae (spaces).  They do not form in the endometrium or in the inner cell mass.  Although spaces or cavities form in the extraembryonic mesoderm, they are not called lacunae and they do not form lacunar networks.  These extraembryonic coelomic spaces become confluent to form the extraembryonic coelom.

8.  C  Ectopic or extrauterine pregnancies usually occur in the ampulla of the uterine tube.  They are related to factors delaying or preventing passage of the morula to the uterus.  Tubal rupture may be followed by early expulsion of a tubal pregnancy and secondary implantation of the blastocyst in the ovary or abdomen.  Ectopic pregnancies, other than in the tube, are rare.  Cervical implantations are not ectopic (outside the uterus), but they are abnormal.  Cervical implantations, usually in the superior part of the cervix, are uncommon.  However, cervical pregnancy is a serious complication of pregnancy because the placenta firmly attaches to the muscles of the cervix.

9.  C  The stratum spongiosum of the endometrium is not directly involved with early implantation.  It does become involved with formation of the placenta later in pregnancy.  The decidual reaction is the series of changes occurring in the endometrium that result from implantation.  It is believed that the blastocyst produces hormone-like substances which cause the decidual changes.  Progesterone produced by the corpus luteum is the hormone believed to control implantation.  Invasion of the endometrium by the syncytiotrophoblast is the most striking event occurring during implantation.  The trophoblast produces proteolytic enzymes which erode the epithelial cells of the endometrium and its connective tissues, glands, and blood vessels.

10.  B  The amniotic cavity appears as a space between the trophoblast and the inner cell mass.  Attachment of the blastocyst to the endometrium usually occurs at the embryonic pole, hence this area is sometimes called the polar trophoblast.  The amniotic cavity does not develop between the extraembryonic mesoderm (or the connecting stalk) and the trophoblast.

# M U L T I - C O M P L E T I O N   Q U E S T I O N S

DIRECTIONS:  In each of the following questions or incomplete statements ONE OR MORE of the completions is correct.  At the lower right of each question, circle A if 1, 2, and 3 are correct; B if 1 and 3 are correct; C if 2 and 4 are correct; D if only 4 is correct; and E if all are correct.

1.  Ectopic implantations may occur in the

    1.  lower uterine segment
    2.  uterine tube
    3.  cervix
    4.  peritoneal cavity                    A B C D E

| A | B | C | D | E |
|---|---|---|---|---|
| 1,2,3 | 1,3 | 2,4 | only 4 | all correct |

2.  Implantation of the blastocyst

  1. is mainly controlled by progesterone
  2. does not occur if the zona pellucida persists
  3. begins at the end of the first week
  4. ends during the second week of development          A B C D E

3.  Important features of the second week of development are the formation of the

  1. extraembryonic mesoderm
  2. primary chorionic villi
  3. amniotic cavity
  4. primitive streak          A B C D E

4.  The part of the 13-day blastocyst which forms the embryo

  1. lies between the amniotic cavity and the yolk sac
  2. also contributes to the roof of the yolk sac
  3. is composed of two primary germ layers
  4. also gives rise to the amnion          A B C D E

5.  During implantation the blastocyst

  1. sinks into the compact layer of the endometrium
  2. initially attaches to the endometrial epithelium at its abembryonic pole
  3. usually implants in the posterior wall of the body of the uterus
  4. has little effect on the endometrial tissues          A B C D E

6.  Criteria used for identification of a section of an 8-day blastocyst are:

  1. The trophoblast at its abembryonic pole consists of a thin layer of flattened cells.
  2. The syncytiotrophoblast at the embryonic pole consists of a thick multinucleated mass.
  3. It is partially embedded in the compact layer of the endometrium.
  4. The inner cell mass is composed of two layers.          A B C D E

7.  Features of the 10- to 12-day blastocyst include:

  1. It is completely embedded in the endometrial stroma.
  2. A closing plug is visible in the endometrial epithelium.
  3. The lacunae in the syncytiotrophoblast are confluent.
  4. Blood from the blood islands on the yolk sac enters the lacunar networks.          A B C D E

23

Clinically Oriented Embryology

| A | B | C | D | E |
|---|---|---|---|---|
| 1,2,3 | 1,3 | 2,4 | only 4 | all correct |

8. By the end of the second week of human development,

   1. primary chorionic villi are usually present
   2. the extraembryonic coelom completely surrounds the amnion and yolk sac
   3. the extraembryonic coelom consists of a large cavity
   4. the corpus luteum has reached its maximum development     A B C D E

9. Correct statements about the chorionic sac include:

   1. It contains the conceptus.
   2. The chorion forms its wall.
   3. It develops poorly in ectopic pregnancies.
   4. Its wall consists of mesoderm and trophoblast.     A B C D E

10. In the 13-day blastocyst, the extraembryonic mesoderm is

   1. divided into two layers by coelom
   2. the third germ layer to form
   3. derived from the cytotrophoblast
   4. derived from the primitive streak     A B C D E

11. In the 14-day blastocyst, the prochordal plate

   1. is a circular area of columnar cells
   2. indicates the future site of the allantois
   3. appears in the future cranial region of the embryo
   4. appears as a thickened area on the floor of the amniotic cavity     A B C D E

12. Characteristics of the decidual reaction include:

   1. The endometrial stromal cells around the conceptus enlarge.
   2. The reaction initially occurs around the implantation site.
   3. The highly modified stromal cells are called decidual cells.
   4. Decidual cells are located in the stratum compactum.     A B C D E

======================== ANSWERS, NOTES, AND EXPLANATIONS ========================

1. **C**  **2 and 4 are correct.** 'Ectopic' implies extrauterine, or outside the uterus. The lower uterine segment and the cervix are abnormal sites of implantation in the uterus. The blastocyst usually implants on the posterior

24

wall slightly more frequently than on the anterior wall of the uterus, inferior to the entrance of the uterine tubes. The most common site of ectopic pregnancy is in the ampulla of the uterine tube. Less commonly the blastocyst implants in other parts of the tube. Following expulsion from the tube, a blastocyst may implant on the peritoneum in the abdomen.

2. E  All are correct.  Implantation begins on day six and is essentially completed by day 10.  Implantation is mainly controlled by progesterone produced by the corpus luteum.  The corpus luteum of pregnancy is maintained by hCG (human chorionic gonadotropin), a hormone much like LH, which is produced by the syncytiotrophoblast.

3. A  1, 2, and 3 are correct.  The primitive streak is not recognizable until the beginning of the third week.  Other important features of the second week not listed are the rapid proliferation and differentiation of the trophoblast and development of the primitive uteroplacental circulation.

4. A  1, 2, and 3 are correct.  The embryonic disc gives rise to the embryo;  it lies between the yolk sac and the amniotic cavity.  The hypoblast of the embryonic disc forms the roof of the yolk sac.  Later this layer becomes endoderm and is folded into the embryo and forms the epithelial lining of the primitive gut.  The amnion is derived from amnioblasts that arise from the cytotrophoblast.  It is continuous with the epiblast at the periphery of the embryonic disc.

5. B  1 and 3 are correct.  The blastocyst implants in the compact layer of the endometrium, slightly more frequently on its posterior than its anterior wall.  It may implant near the internal ostium (os), or opening, of the uterus.  This results in the condition of placenta previa (the placenta covers or adjoins the internal ostium causing obstetrical complications).  Implantation in the cervix may also occur.  As the placenta develops and increases in size, the chorionic villi extend into the spongy layer of the endometrium.  The trophoblast over the inner cell mass, i.e., at the embryonic pole, is usually the first site of attachment of the blastocyst to the endometrium.  During implantation, the endometrium is exposed to the activities of the trophoblast, which appears to produce substances that exert a profound effect on the endometrium.  Although initially confined to the area immediately around the conceptus, the decidual reaction soon spreads throughout the endometrium.

6. E  All are correct.  These criteria enable one to identify a section of endometrium containing an 8-day blastocyst.  The free part of the blastocyst, projecting into the uterine cavity, consists of a thin layer of cytotrophoblast cells.

7. A  1, 2, and 3 are correct.  Blood and blood vessels do not appear in the wall of the yolk sac until the third week.  This primitive blood flows into the embryo, but does not enter the lacunar networks.  Maternal blood from eroded sinusoids seeps into the lacunar networks and forms the primitive uteroplacental circulation.  The closing plug is usually visible in the epithelium covering the 10- to 11-day blastocyst, but by the twelfth day, the

regenerated endometrial epithelium covers over the blastocyst and the closing plug is inconspicuous.

8. B  <u>1 and 3 are correct</u>.  The development of primary chorionic villi is a main feature of the second week of development.  The extraembryonic coelom is a large cavity that surrounds the amnion and yolk sac, <u>except</u> where the amnion and embryonic disc are attached to the wall of the chorionic sac by the connecting stalk (future umbilical cord).  The corpus luteum of pregnancy continues to grow.  By the end of the third month it is usually one-third to one-half of the total size of the ovary.

9. C  <u>2 and 4 are correct</u>.  The wall of the chorionic sac is composed of the chorion, consisting of the two layers of trophoblast (cytotrophoblast and syncytiotrophobast), which is lined by a layer of extraembryonic somatic mesoderm.  It is not correct to say that the chorion contains the conceptus because the chorionic sac is a part of the conceptus (i.e., the term means the embryo and its membranes).  It is correct to say that the chorionic sac contains the embryo (embryonic disc) and its associated amniotic and yolk sacs suspended within the chorionic sac by the connecting stalk.  The chorionic sac develops well when implantation occurs outside the uterus.  Of course the optimum site for development of the blastocyst is in the endometrium.  Ectopic pregnancy usually leads to expulsion of the conceptus and death of the embryo during the fifth to sixth week.

10. B  <u>1 and 3 are correct</u>.  This mesoderm is extraembryonic, i.e., outside the embryo, and does not form embryonic tissues.  The primitive streak is not visible in the 13-day blastocyst.  The third primary germ layer, intra-embryonic mesoderm, is derived from the primitive streak as it forms during the third week.

11. B  <u>1 and 3 are correct</u>.  The prochordal plate appears on the ventral surface of the future cranial end of the embryonic disc as a thickened, circular area of hypoblast.  It indicates the future cranial region of the embryo and the future site of the mouth.  It appears at the cranial end of the roof of the yolk sac and its presence confers bilateral symmetry on the embryonic disc because the right and left sides of the embryonic disc are not identifiable.

12. E  <u>All are correct</u>.  The cellular, vascular, and glandular alterations occurring during the decidual reaction are believed to result from substances produced by the syncytiotrophoblast.  The nature of these substances is not clearly understood, but they are able to destroy endometrial cells.  The degenerated cells are ingested by the trophoblast and the materials are utilized for nourishment.  The decidual reaction is at first confined to the area around the implantation site, but the changes soon spread through the endometrium.

# FIVE-CHOICE ASSOCIATION QUESTIONS

DIRECTIONS: Each group of questions below consists of a numbered list of descriptive words or phrases accompanied by a diagram with certain parts indicated by letters, or by a list of lettered headings. For each numbered word or phrase, SELECT THE LETTERED PART OR HEADING that matches it correctly. Then insert the letter in the space to the right of the appropriate number. Sometimes more than one numbered word or phrase may be correctly matched to the same lettered part or heading.

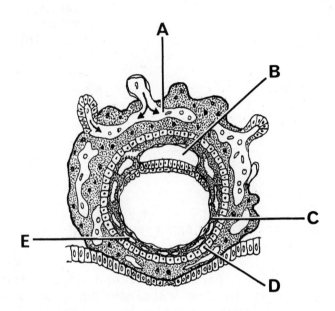

| | | |
|---|---|---|
| 1. E | Extraembryonic coelom | |
| — 2. A | Contains embryotroph | |
| 3. D | Cytotrophoblast | |
| 4. A | Lacunar network | |
| 5. B | Epiblast forms its floor | |

A. Corpus luteum
B. Zona pellucida
C. Prochordal plate
D. Ectopic implantation
E. Chorionic sac

| | |
|---|---|
| 6. D | Frequently occurs in the uterine tube |
| 7. C | Develops as a localized thickening of the hypoblast |
| 8. A | Develops from a ruptured ovarian follicle |
| 9. B | Surrounds the embryo and its amnion and yolk sac |
| 10. A | Enlarges greatly if implantation of a blastocyst occurs |

## ASSOCIATION QUESTIONS

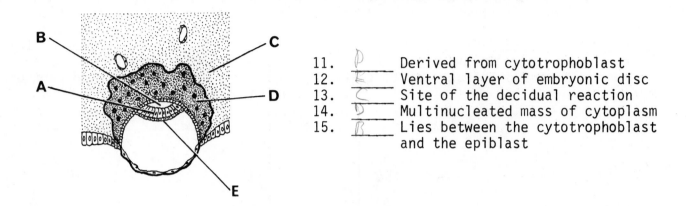

11. _D_____ Derived from cytotrophoblast
12. _E_____ Ventral layer of embryonic disc
13. _C_____ Site of the decidual reaction
14. _D_____ Multinucleated mass of cytoplasm
15. _B_____ Lies between the cytotrophoblast
and the epiblast

======================= ANSWERS, NOTES, AND EXPLANATIONS ========================

1.  E  The extraembryonic coelom, part of which is indicated in the diagram, consists of isolated spaces in the extraembryonic mesoderm. Later these spaces fuse or coalesce to form a single large cavity, known as the extraembryonic coelom.

2.  A  The lacunar networks (future intervillous spaces) contain a nutrient material known as embryotroph. It is required by the embryo for growth and differentiation. Embryotroph consists of maternal blood, degenerated decidual cells, blood vessels, and glandular tissue.

3.  D  The cytotrophoblast is the inner layer of the trophoblast. It gives rise to: (1) the outer layer of trophoblast (syncytiotrophoblast); (2) amnioblasts (cells that form the amnion); (3) the extraembryonic mesoderm. The cytotrophoblast, as the prefix 'cyto' implies, is a cellular layer.

4.  A  The lacunar networks form by coalescence of spaces in the syncytiotrophoblast. As the maternal sinusoids are eroded, blood seeps into these networks. Nutrients in the embryotroph diffuse through the two layers of trophoblast and pass to the embryo via the extraembryonic coelom.

5.  B  The floor of the amniotic cavity consists of embryonic epiblast. The amnion enclosing the amniotic cavity is attached to the epiblast of the embryonic disc. Initially some amniotic fluid may be secreted by the amniotic cells, but most of it is derived from the maternal blood.

6.  D  Ectopic implantations usually occur in the uterine tube, most frequently in the ampulla where fertilization normally occurs. Other sites of ectopic (outside the uterus) implantations are in the ovary and on the abdominal peritoneum.

7.  C  The prochordal plate indicates the future cranial end of the embryo and the future site of the mouth. It is a circular area that is firmly adherent to the overlying embryonic epiblast. It is an important landmark in the early embryo and seems to serve as an organizer of the cranial region of the embryo.

8.  A  The corpus luteum develops from the ovarian follicle following ovulation. Under the influence of LH produced by the hypophysis (anterior pituitary gland), the ruptured follicle develops into a glandular structure. At ovulation the walls of the follicle collapse and, with cells of the theca folliculi, form the corpus luteum. The corpus luteum is an important source of progesterone for about four months. After this, the placenta is the major producer of this hormone.

9.  E  The chorion forms a chorionic sac from the wall of which the embryo, its amnion, and its yolk sac are suspended by the connecting stalk. The chorion gives rise to the embryonic part of the placenta. The maternal part of the placenta develops from the endometrium (decidua basalis).

10. A  If an ovum is fertilized and the blastocyst implants, the corpus luteum enlarges to form a corpus luteum of pregnancy and increases its production of progesterone. This hormone is necessary for the maintenance of pregnancy. The corpus luteum is an important source of progesterone during the first trimester (three months); it also produces estrogen. In later pregnancy, these hormones are produced by the placenta.

11. D  The syncytiotrophoblast is derived from the cytotrophoblast. Cells of the cytotrophoblast divide mitotically and some of these cells move outward where they fuse with and become part of the increasing mass of syncytiotrophoblast. The syncytiotrophoblast produces human chorionic gonadotropin which acts like LH in maintaining the corpus luteum. Later it also produces other hormones.

12. E  The hypoblast (primitive endoderm) forms the ventral layer of the embryonic disc. It is the primordium of the endoderm of the embryo. It is first recognizable on the ventral surface of the inner cell mass about seven days after fertilization.

13. C  The stroma (connective tissue) in the compact layer of the endometrium in the region of the implanting blastocyst is the site of cellular and other changes known as the decidual reaction. The enlarged cells, called decidual cells, contain large amounts of glycogen and lipids that provide nourishment for the embryo.

14. D  The syncytiotrophoblast is a multinucleated protoplasmic mass derived by division of cytotrophoblast cells. This layer is devoid of cell boundaries. The syncytiotrophoblast is actively involved during implantation and produces substances which cause the decidual reaction. Later this layer produces two protein hormones and two steroid hormones.

15.   B   The amniotic cavity lies between the cytotrophoblast at the embryonic pole and the embryonic epiblast of the embryonic disc.  Cells from the cytotrophoblast (amnioblasts) soon form a thin roof over this cavity called the amnion.  It is continuous with the epiblast of the embryonic disc.

_____

NOTES:

# FORMATION OF THE TRILAMINAR EMBRYO

The Third Week

## O B J E C T I V E S

BE ABLE TO:

_____

o   Describe the formation and growth of the primitive streak, using simple diagrams to illustrate formation of the intraembryonic mesoderm and the trilaminar embryo.

o   Define: primitive knot, primitive groove, and primitive pit.

o   Trace the development of the notochord, using simple diagrammatic sections of 3-week embryos.

o   Define: notochordal process, notochordal canal, and notochordal plate.

o   Give an account of the development of the neural tube using simple sketches.

o   Define: neural plate, neural groove, neural folds, and neural crest.

o   Illustrate, with simple sketches, the development of the following: somites, paraxial mesoderm, intermediate mesoderm, lateral mesoderm, intraembryonic coelom, tertiary villi, blood and blood vessels.

o   Construct and label diagrams showing the early development of the cardiovascular system and the sites of blood formation.

o   Define: angioblasts and blood islands.

o   Write brief notes on the allantois, oropharyngeal membrane, and cloacal membrane.

_____

## F I V E - C H O I C E   C O M P L E T I O N   Q U E S T I O N S

DIRECTIONS:  Each of the following statements or questions is followed by five suggested responses or completions.  SELECT THE ONE BEST ANSWER in each case and then circle the appropriate letter at the right of each question.

1.   Human chorionic gonadotropin (hGC) is a hormone produced by the

   A.  syncytiotrophoblast              D.  theca folliculi
   B.  anterior pituitary gland         E.  hypophysis cerebri
   C.  corpus luteum of pregnancy
                                                          A B C D E

31

## SELECT THE ONE BEST ANSWER

2.  The primitive streak first appears at the beginning of the _____ week.

    A.  first                   D.  fourth
    B.  second                  E.  fifth
    C.  third                                       A B C D E

3.  The notochordal process lengthens by migration of cells from the

    A.  notochord               D.  primitive knot
    B.  primitive streak        E.  neural plate
    C.  notochordal plate                           A B C D E

4.  The notochordal plate infolds to form the

    A.  neural tube             D.  notochordal canal
    B.  neurenteric canal       E.  notochord
    C.  notochordal process                         A B C D E

5.  During the third week the neurenteric canal connects the amniotic
    cavity and the

    A.  allantois
    B.  neural tube
    C.  caudal neuropore
    D.  yolk sac
    E.  chorionic cavity                            A B C D E

6.  The intraembryonic coelom located cranial to the oropharyngeal
    membrane becomes the

    A.  mouth cavity            D.  pharyngeal cavity
    B.  stomodeum               E.  pleural cavity
    C.  pericardial cavity                          A B C D E

7.  The cloacal membrane consists of

    A.  embryonic endoderm, mesoderm, and ectoderm
    B.  a circular area of endoderm fused to embryonic mesoderm
    C.  endoderm of the roof of the yolk sac and embryonic ectoderm
    D.  the prochordal plate and the overlying embryonic ectoderm
    E.  extraembryonic layers of the mesoderm       A B C D E

8.  The specialized group of mesenchymal cells which aggregate to
    form blood islands are called

    A.  hemoblasts              D.  mesoblasts
    B.  angioblasts             E.  none of the above
    C.  fibroblasts                                 A B C D E

SELECT THE ONE BEST ANSWER

9.  The primitive blood cells of the three-week embryo first begin
    to form

    A.  at 19 to 20 days          D.  in the liver
    B.  in the embryonic disc     E.  in the allantois
    C.  on the yolk sac                              A B C D E

======================= ANSWERS, NOTES, AND EXPLANATIONS =========================

1.  A   It is generally believed that the syncytiotrophoblast layer of the
    trophoblast produces human chorionic gonadotropic (hCG), and that this
    hormone stimulates the corpus luteum of pregnancy to increase in size and to
    continue producing hormones.  Progestrone produced by the corpus luteum is
    necessary for maintenance of pregnancy during the early months.  Thereafter
    progesterone is produced by the syncytiotrophoblast of the placenta.

2.  C  The primitive streak usually appears in 15-day-old embryos, i.e., at the
    beginning of the third week.  Cells from the primitive streak pass between
    the ectoderm and endoderm and form the third germ layer (mesoderm).

3.  D  If you chose B, the primitive streak, you are partly right because the
    primitive knot is the cranial end of the primitive streak.  However, D is the
    better answer.  Cells migrate cranially from the primitive knot to form a
    midline cord known as the notochordal process.  The primitive knot is a
    thickening of the epiblast at the cranial end of the primitive streak.  In
    addition to forming the notochordal process, cells from the primitive knot
    also form intraembryonic mesoderm.

4.  E  The notochordal plate infolds to form the notochord.  The primordium of
    the notochord is the notochordal process.  The notochordal canal develops in
    the notochordal process as the primitive pit invaginates into it.

5.  D  The neurenteric canal is associated with late stages of notochord develop-
    ment.  It represents the part of the notochordal canal that does not dis-
    appear when the floor of the notochordal process degenerates.  The neuren-
    teric canal connects the amniotic cavity and the yolk sac.  It usually
    disappears when the notochord is fully developed (about 5 weeks).  In most
    cases the brief existence of the canal is of no significance.

6.  C  The pericardial cavity and the developing heart are carried ventrally with
    the head fold as the brain grows rapidly during the fourth week.  The
    pericardial cavity forms by confluence of small isolated spaces in the
    cardiogenic (heart-forming) mesoderm which lies cranial to the oropharyngeal
    membrane.

7.  C  The cloacal membrane is the circular bilaminar area where the embryonic
    endoderm of the roof of the yolk sac contacts and fuses with the overlying
    embryonic ectoderm caudal to the primitive streak.  There is no mesoderm

between the two layers composing the cloacal membrane. The area where the prochordal plate fuses with the overlying ectoderm is called the oropharyngeal membrane.

8. B Angioblasts are specialized mesenchymal cells that give rise to blood and to the vascular and lymphatic systems. Fibroblasts are connective tissue cells which form fibrous tissues in the body. Hemoblasts are blood cells that are usually called hemocytoblasts.

9. C Primitive blood first forms in the extraembryonic mesoderm associated with the yolk sac, the allantois, and the connecting stalk at 15 to 16 days. Blood formation does not begin in the embryo until the sixth week, when it forms in the liver. Hence the blood in the three-week embryo forms in the extraembryonic membranes and flows into the cardiovascular system as the embryonic vessels form.

# MULTI-COMPLETION QUESTIONS

DIRECTIONS: In each of the following questions or incomplete statements ONE OR MORE of the completions is correct. At the lower right of each question, circle A if 1, 2, and 3 are correct; B if 1 and 3 are correct; C if 2 and 4 are correct; D if only 4 is correct; and E if all are correct.

1. Tertiary chorionic villi contain a core of

   1. mesenchymal cells
   2. syncytiotrophoblast
   3. blood capillaries
   4. decidual cells                          A B C D E

2. The human trilaminar embryonic disc is

   1. formed during the early part of the third week
   2. composed of three primary germ layers
   3. initially flat and wide at its cranial end
   4. characterized by the primitive streak caudally          A B C D E

3. Intraembryonic mesenchyme

   1. separates the ectoderm and endoderm at the cloacal membrane
   2. forms a 'packing tissue' around developing organs
   3. surrounds the umbilical vessels in the connecting stalk
   4. is derived from the third germ layer (i.e., mesoderm)      A B C D E

4. The paired somites

   1. first appear at the end of the third week
   2. are formed by division of the paraxial mesoderm
   3. initially form at the cranial end of the notochord
   4. usually cease forming by the end of the fourth week       A B C D E

| A | B | C | D | E |
|---|---|---|---|---|
| 1,2,3 | 1,3 | 2,4 | only 4 | all correct |

5. The paraxial mesoderm

    1. appears as a longitudinal column on each side of the
notochordal process
    2. is continuous medially with the intermediate mesoderm
    3. gives rise to all somites developing during the embry-
onic period
    4. is separated from the intermediate mesoderm by
lateral mesoderm                           A B C D E

6. The oropharyngeal membrane is

    1. composed of ectoderm and endoderm
    2. located at the future site of the mouth
    3. associated with the cranial end of the notochord
    4. a trilaminar membrane situated cranial to the notochord    A B C D E

7. Structures involved in formation of the notochord include the

    1. primitive streak           3. embryonic mesoderm
    2. notochordal plate          4. primitive pit        A B C D E

8. The cloacal membrane is

    1. a trilaminar membrane
    2. composed of fused layers of ectoderm and endoderm
    3. closely associated with the primitive knot
    4. located between the primitive streak and the connect-
ing stalk                                  A B C D E

9. Extraembryonic somatic mesoderm

    1. is in contact with the cytotrophoblast of the chorion
    2. together with the overlying ectoderm forms the body wall
    3. covers the amnion and is continuous with the lateral
mesoderm
    4. is involved in formation of the cranial somites       A B C D E

10. Correct statements concerning early development of the
central nervous system include:

    1. As the primitive streak develops, the embryonic ectoderm
over it thickens to form the neural plate.
    2. The neural plate is composed of neuroectoderm and is
thicker than the surface ectoderm.
    3. By the middle of the third week the neural folds have
begun to fuse caudally.
    4. Most of the neural tube gives rise to the spinal cord.    A B C D E

| A | B | C | D | E |
|---|---|---|---|---|
| 1,2,3 | 1,3 | 2,4 | only 4 | all correct |

11. The median cellular cord called the notochord

    1. forms the embryonic basis of the axial skeleton
    2. initially forms cranially and develops caudally as
       the embryo grows
    3. comes into contact with the caudal edge of the oro-
       pharyngeal membrane
    4. lies in the median plane between the roof of the yolk
       sac and the embryonic ectoderm                        A B C D E

12. Remnants of the primitive streak are most likely to

    1. give rise to tumors in males
    2. appear in the sacrococcygeal region
    3. give rise to chordomas in females
    4. give rise to a sacrococcygeal teratoma                 A B C D E


=====================  ANSWERS, NOTES, AND EXPLANATIONS  =======================

1. B  1 and 3 are correct.  The mesenchymal core of primitive villi becomes the
   loose connective tissue of the chorionic villi of the mature placenta.
   Development of blood capillaries containing primitive plasma and blood cells
   is the criterion used to identify tertiary villi.  The syncytiotrophoblast
   forms the external layer of the wall of the villus; it is not contained within the wall of the villus.  Decidual cells are large, specialized endometrial stromal cells.

2. E  All are correct.  The trilaminar embryonic disc begins to form early in
   the third week and is composed of three term layers (ectoderm, mesoderm, and
   endoderm).  The primitive streak is a characteristic feature of the dorsal
   surface of the embryonic disc during the third week.

3. C  2 and 4 are correct.  The mesenchyme in the embryo acts as a 'packing
   tissue, around developing structures (e.g., the neural tube).  It gives rise
   to connective tissue and muscles.  There is no mesenchyme, or any other
   tissue, between the ectoderm and the endoderm at the cloacal membrane.  The
   mesenchyme in the connecting stalk is derived from extraembryonic mesoderm.

4. A  1, 2, and 3 are correct.  The somites begin to appear around the end of
   the third week, a short distance caudal to the cranial tip of the notochord.
   Successive somites are formed by division and differentiation of the paraxial
   mesoderm.  Each new pair of somites lies immediately caudal to the previously
   formed pair.  The somites are still forming rapidly at the end of the fourth
   week, but they are usually all formed by the end of the fifth week.  The
   somites form one of the embryo's most characteristic features.  Hence the
   number present is often used to determine the age of an aborted embryo.

5.  B  1 and 3 are correct.  The paraxial mesoderm appears as a longitudinal column on each side of the median plane.  Beginning cranially, it divides and differentiates into somites.  It is continuous laterally with the intermediate mesoderm which separates it from the lateral mesoderm.

6.  A  1, 2, and 3 are correct.  The oropharyngeal membrane is bilaminar, composed of ectoderm and endoderm, and lies cranial to the notochord.  During the fourth week it ruptures, bringing the primitive oral cavity into communication with the primitive pharynx.  It is composed of ectoderm and endoderm; it is not trilaminar (composed of three layers).

7.  E  All are correct.  The notochord arises from the notochordal process which develops from the mesenchymal cells arising from the primitive knot of the primitive streak.  The primitive pit in the primitive knot extends into the notochordal process to form the notochordal canal.  The endoderm forming the roof of the yolk sac breaks down where it is fused with the notochordal process, allowing communication between the yolk sac and the amniotic cavity via the neurenteric canal.  The notochordal plate infolds to form the notochord.

8.  C  2 and 4 are correct.  The cloacal membrane is bilaminar (composed of ectoderm and endoderm), and lies caudal to the primitive streak, near the connecting stalk.  It is not associated with the primitive knot which is located at the cranial end of the primitive streak.

9.  B  1 and 3 are correct.  The extraembryonic somatic mesoderm is located outside the embryo, lining the chorion and forming an external covering for the amnion.  It is continuous with the embryonic somatic mesoderm that lines the body wall.  The embryonic somatic mesoderm and the embryonic ectoderm form the body wall (embryonic somatopleure).

10.  C  2 and 4 are correct.  The ectoderm of the neural plate, called neuroectoderm, is thick compared to the surface ectoderm (the source of the epidermis).  The ectoderm over the developing notochord thickens to form the neural plate.  The cranial end of the neural tube forms the brain and the large caudal part gives rise to the spinal cord.  The neural folds begin to fuse during the early part of the fourth week to form the neural tube.

11.  E  All are correct.  The notochord forms the only skeleton in lower chordates, e.g., the Amphioxus.  The notochord of human embryos degenerates after the vertebral body forms around it.  Between the vertebrae, the notochord persists and gives rise to the nucleus pulposus of the intervertebral disc.

12.  C  2 and 4 are correct.  Remnants of the primitive streak (one kind of embryonic cell rest) may persist and give rise to teratomas in the sacrococcygeal region.  These tumors are much more common in females and are usually benign in newborn infants.  Chordomas are believed to arise from remnants of the notochord in the bodies of vertebrae.  Teratomas are located in the region of the coccyx or inferior part of the sacrum, and probably are derived from cells of the primitive knot.  Interestingly, there is a significant increase in the incidence of twinning in families of infants with sacrococcygeal tumors.  Most of these tumors are apparent at birth, usually presenting as a mass at the tip of the coccyx.  Large ones extend postero-inferiorly and fill one buttock as far anteriorly as the anus.  Internally

they often occupy the entire hollow of the sacrum and push the rectum anteriorly. Sacrococcygeal teratomas demonstrate malignant changes more often than do teratomas in other locations.

## F I V E - C H O I C E   A S S O C I A T I O N   Q U E S T I O N S

DIRECTIONS: Each group of questions below consists of a numbered list of descriptive words or phrases accompanied by a diagram with certain parts indicated by letters, or by a list of lettered headings. For each numbered word or phrase, SELECT THE LETTERED PART OR HEADING that matches it correctly. Then insert the letter in the space to the right of the appropriate number. Sometimes more than one numbered word or phrase may be correctly matched to the same lettered part or heading.

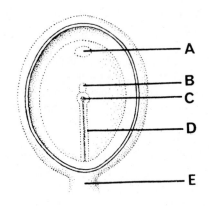

1. _B_ Notochordal process
2. _A_ Site of the prochordal plate
3. _D_ Gives rise to mesoderm
4. _A_ Ventral layer of the oropharyngeal membrane
5. _C_ Primitive pit

A. Allantois
B. Primitive streak
C. Notochord
D. Blood island
E. Neural plate

6. _D_ Aggregation of angioblasts
7. _A_ Diverticulum of the yolk sac
8. _C_ Induces embryonic ectoderm to thicken
9. _C_ Forms the basis of the axial skeleton
10. _E_ Gives rise to the brain and spinal cord
11. _B_ Source of mesenchyme
12. _A_ Rudimentary structure
13. _D_ Appears in an extraembryonic membrane

ASSOCIATION QUESTIONS

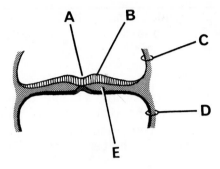

14. _C_____ Wall of the amniotic sac
15. _A_____ Neural groove
16. _E_____ Derived from the primitive streak
17. _B_____ Embryonic ectoderm

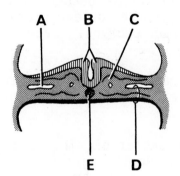

18. _C_____ Derived from paraxial mesoderm
19. _E_____ Derived from the notochordal process
20. _A_____ Gives rise to an adult body cavity
21. _D_____ Splanchnopleure
22. _B_____ Fusing to form the neural tube

======================= ANSWERS, NOTES, AND EXPLANATIONS =========================

1.  B  The notochordal process is a rod-shaped structure composed of cells derived from the primitive knot. It is the primordium of the notochord, a cellular structure which defines the primitive axis of the embryo.

2.  A  The site of the prochordal plate is indicated in the drawing by a dotted oval to indicate that it is not visible from the dorsal surface of the embryonic disc. The prochordal plate is a circular area of thickened embryonic endoderm in the cranial part of the roof of the yolk sac. The prochordal plate, together with the overlying embryonic ectoderm later constitutes the oropharyngeal membrane.

3.    D  The primitive streak, a linear band, gives rise to mesoderm mainly during the third week.  As the mesoderm is produced by the primitive streak, it extends laterally until it becomes continuous with the extraembryonic mesoderm on the amnion and yolk sac.  The intraembryonic mesoderm becomes thickened on each side of the embryonic axis to form two longitudinal columns of paraxial mesoderm.

4.    A  The ventral layer of the bilaminar oropharyngeal membrane is the prochordal plate; the dorsal layer is embryonic ectoderm.  This membrane ruptures during the fourth week bringing the primitive oral cavity into communication with the primitive pharynx.

5.    C  The primitive pit is a depression in the primitive knot at the cranial end of the primitive streak.  It extends into the notochordal process and forms the notochordal canal.  Thus it is the entrance to the notochordal canal.  It later forms the opening of the neurenteric canal which temporarily connects the amniotic cavity with the yolk sac.

6.    D  Mesenchymal cells known as angioblasts aggregate to form isolated masses and cords, known as blood islands.  These masses give rise to primitive plasma, blood cells, and blood vessels.  Blood islands form first in the yolk sac, chorion, allantois and connecting stalk, but they develop in the embryo about two days later.

7.    A  The allantois is a vestigial structure which later becomes the urachus (median umbilical ligament).  It serves as a reservoir for excretory products in some species, but it is nonfunctional in human embryos.  Later, however, its blood vessels become the umbilical vessels.

8.    C  The developing notochord and the adjacent paraxial mesoderm are thought to produce inductive substances which stimulate development of the neural plate from the overlying embryonic ectoderm.

9.    C  The notochord forms the basis of the axial skeleton.  The vertebrae develop around it and then it degenerates.  In between the vertebrae, the notochord gives rise to the nucleus pulposus of the intervertebral disc.

10.   E  The neural plate is a thickened area of ectoderm (neuroectoderm) overlying and extending on each side of the notochord.  The neural plate sinks in to form a neural groove.  In later development, the neural folds meet dorsally to form the neural tube.  The cranial part of neural tube gives rise to the brain and the larger remaining part forms the spinal cord.  The notochord and paraxial mesoderm produce inductive substances which stimulate or induce the overlying ectoderm to thicken and form the neural plate.

11.   B  The primitive streak produces mesoderm which gives rise to mesenchyme (embryonic connective tissue).  Mesenchyme forms a 'packing tissue' around developing organs and gives rise to connective tissues and muscles.

12.   A  The allantois is a rudimentary structure.  Although the allantois does not

function in human embryos, it is important because blood formation occurs in its walls, and its blood vessels become the umbilical vessels.

13. D   The blood islands first appear in the walls of the yolk sac, the allantois, and connecting stalk. These extraembryonic membranes are derived from the zygote, but they are not part of the embryo. The roof of the yolk sac becomes incorporated into the embryo during the fourth week and forms the primitive gut. Blood islands form in the embryo about two days after they appear on the yolk sac.

14. C   The amnion encloses the amniotic cavity, forming an amniotic sac. It contains fluid which bathes the embryonic disc forming its floor. The wall of this sac consists of an inner epithelial layer of cells covered externally by extraembryonic somatic mesoderm.

15. A   The neural groove forms as the neural plate invaginates to form a neural fold on each side. The folds later fuse to form the neural tube, the primordium of the central nervous system (brain and spinal cord). The ectoderm lateral to the folds, known as surface ectoderm, will give rise to the epidermis of the skin.

16. E   The intraembryonic mesoderm is derived from the primitive streak. The primitive streak produces mesoderm rapidly during the third and fourth weeks.

17. B   The embryonic ectoderm in the region indicated forms a neural fold. The neural folds soon fuse converting the neural plate into the neural tube, the primordium of the central nervous system (brain and spinal cord).

18. C   The somites are paired cubical masses derived by division or segmentation of the paraxial mesoderm. The first pair of somites is formed a short distance caudal to the tip of the notochord and successive somites are progressively formed from paraxial mesoderm. Most somites appear between days 20 and 30; they give rise to the axial skeleton and its associated musculature.

19. E   The notochord arises from the notochordal process. The notochord is a cellular rod that defines the primitive axis of the embryo. Mesenchymal cells from the somites later surround it and give rise to the mesenchymal bodies of the vertebrate. The notochord within the developing vertebrae later degenerates.

20. A   The intraembryonic coelom in the area indicated will give rise to part of the peritoneal cavity. The coelom appears here as a space within the lateral mesoderm, splitting it into somatic and splanchnic layers. The transverse section is cut through the caudal region of the lateral extensions of the horseshoe-shaped body cavity or coelom.

21. D   The embryonic splanchnopleure is composed of splanchnic mesoderm and endoderm, and represents the future wall of the primitive gut. The endoderm gives rise to the epithelium and glands of the digestive tract; the mesoderm gives rise to its muscular and fibrous elements.

22. **B** The neural folds are fusing to form the neural tube, the primordium of the brain and spinal cord. These folds form as the neural plate invaginates along its central axis to form a neural groove with neural folds on each side.

---

NOTES:

# FORMATION OF BASIC ORGANS AND SYSTEMS

The Fourth to Eighth Weeks

## O B J E C T I V E S

BE ABLE TO:

_____

o    Draw and label simple sketches showing the main developmental
     events of each week during this five-week period.
o    Explain why the fourth to eighth weeks constitute the critical
     period of human development.
o    Define: neuropore, branchial arch, aortic arch, otic pit, lens
     placode, limb bud, and cervical flexure.
o    Estimate the age of embryos traced from drawings in your
     textbook, using the table in your textbook and crown-rump
     measurements.
o    Briefly indicate what each germ layer normally contributes to the
     tissues and organs of the embryo.
o    Discuss induction, using the neural plate and the developing eye
     as examples.
o    Discuss the establishment of general body form resulting from
     folding of the embryo, with special reference to the effect of
     this process on the septum transversum, heart, foregut, midgut,
     allantois, and yolk sac.

_____


## F I V E - C H O I C E   C O M P L E T I O N   Q U E S T I O N S

DIRECTIONS:  Each of the following statements or questions is followed by five
suggested responses or completions.  SELECT THE ONE BEST ANSWER in each case and
then circle the appropriate letter at the right of each question.

1.   All the essential features of external body form of the embryo
     are completed by the end of the _____ week.

     A.   fourth
     B.   sixth
     C.   eighth
     D.   tenth
     E.   twelfth                                              A  B  C  D  E

## SELECT THE ONE BEST ANSWER

2.  During the early part of the fourth week, the rate of growth at the periphery of the embryonic disc fails to keep pace with the rate of growth of the

    A.  yolk sac
    B.  amniotic cavity
    C.  embryonic coelom
    D.  notochordal process
    E.  neural tube

    A B C D E

3.  By the middle of the fourth week, the neural folds at the cranial end of the embryo have begun to develop into the

    A.  neural crest
    B.  spinal cord
    C.  brain
    D.  neural groove
    E.  neural tube

    A B C D E

4.  After folding of the head region, the mesodermal structure lying just caudal to the pericardial cavity is the

    A.  developing heart
    B.  connecting stalk
    C.  primitive streak
    D.  septum transversum
    E.  notochord

    A B C D E

5.  Each of the following structures turn under onto the ventral surface of the embryo during folding of the head <u>except</u> the

    A.  oropharyngeal membrane
    B.  notochord
    C.  heart
    D.  pericardial cavity
    E.  septum transversum

    A B C D E

6.  The terminal dilated part of the hindgut is called the

    A.  allantois
    B.  yolk stalk
    C.  cloaca
    D.  vitelline duct
    E.  cecum

    A B C D E

7.  Each of the following structures is derived from mesoderm <u>except</u>

    A.  muscle
    B.  cartilage
    C.  mesenchyme
    D.  blood vessel
    E.  epidermis

    A B C D E

8.  Which of the following structures is believed to be a primary inductor during organogenesis?

    A.  Somite
    B.  Notochord
    C.  Yolk sac
    D.  Primitive streak
    E.  Lens

    A B C D E

SELECT THE ONE BEST ANSWER

9.  Each of the following is a distinctive characteristic of
    4-week-old embryos <u>except</u>

    A.  somites                    D.  lower limb buds
    B.  hand plates                E.  neuropores
    C.  branchial arches                                A B C D E

10. The most frequently used method for measuring the length of
    5-week-old embryos is

    A.  greatest length            D.  crown-heel length
    B.  standing height            E.  total length
    C.  crown-rump length                               A B C D E

11. The age of the embryo illustrated is _____ weeks.

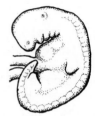

    A.  3
    B.  4
    C.  5
    D.  6
    E.  7                                               A B C D E

======================= ANSWERS, NOTES, AND EXPLANATIONS =======================

1.  C  By the end of the embryonic period (eight weeks), the beginnings of all
    major external and internal structures have developed.  Because of this,
    these five weeks constitute the most critical period of development and the
    time when major developmental disturbances may occur.

2.  E  Because of the rapid growth of the neural tube, the embryo bulges into the
    amniotic cavity and the head and tail regions fold under the cranial and
    caudal parts of the embryonic disc.  Concurrently, marked folding occurs
    along the lateral margins of the disc.

3.  C  By the middle of the fourth week, the neural folds at the center of the
    embryo have started to move together and fuse into the neural tube.  At the
    cranial end of the embryo, the thick neural folds indicate where the brain
    will develop.  By the end of the fourth week, the neural folds in the cranial
    region have fused to form primary brain vesicles which develop into the
    brain.

4.  D  The mesodermal mass known as the septum transversum forms the caudal wall
    of the pericardial cavity.  This mesodermal septum is the primordium of the

central tendon of the diaphragm. After folding of the head, the heart lies dorsal to the pericardial cavity. The primitive streak and the connecting stalk lie considerably caudal to the pericardial cavity.

5. B  The cranial end of the notochord may bend slightly as the forebrain folds ventrally, but the notochord does not turn onto the ventral surface as the other structures do (e.g., the heart).

6. C  Shortly after the caudal part of the yolk sac is incorporated into the embryo as the hindgut, the terminal part of the hindgut dilates to form the cloaca. Its cavity is separated from the amniotic cavity by the cloacal membrane.

7. E  The epidermis is derived from the surface ectoderm. The dermis of the skin is derived from mesoderm, as are all types of connective tissue. The cartilages in the branchial arches are derived from neural crest cells.

8. B  From experiments on lower vertebrates, it is well established that substances produced by the notochordal process and later the notochord, induce the neural plate to form. The lenses appear to function as secondary inductors.

9. B  Hand plates are not visible during the fourth week. They are not distinctive characteristics of the limbs until the fifth week.

10. C  Crown-rump measurements are most commonly taken. Greatest length is used for straight embryos, e.g., during the third week. Crown-heel measurements (standing height) are sometimes used for older embryos, but they are often difficult to make on formalin-fixed embryos because these are difficult to straighten.

11. B  The distinctive characteristics of the four-week embryo (about 28 days) illustrated here are: (1) four branchial arches; (2) a flipper-like upper limb bud; and (3) small lower limb bud.


M U L T I - C O M P L E T I O N   Q U E S T I O N S

DIRECTIONS:  In each of the following questions or incomplete statements ONE OR MORE of the completions is correct. At the lower right of each question, circle A if 1, 2, and 3 are correct; B if 1 and 3 are correct; C if 2 and 4 are correct; D if only 4 is correct; and E if all are correct.


1.  Folding of the embryo in the longitudinal plane results from

    1. rapid growth at the periphery of the embryonic disc
    2. the 'swinging' ventrally of the head and tail regions
    3. incorporation of the cranial part of the yolk sac into the embryo
    4. active growth and development of the neural tube          A B C D E

| A | B | C | D | E |
|---|---|---|---|---|
| 1,2,3 | 1,3 | 2,4 | only 4 | all correct |

2. The dorsal part of the yolk sac is incorporated into the embryo during folding and gives rise to the:

   1. primitive gut           3. midgut
   2. foregut              4. hindgut            A B C D E

3. Structures moving ventrally during folding at the caudal end of the embryo include the

   1. allantois           3. primitive streak
   2. cloacal membrane     4. yolk stalk         A B C D E

4. As the forebrain develops and overhangs the primitive heart, structures turned ventrally by the head fold include the

   1. amnion            3. septum transversum
   2. connecting stalk      4. allantois          A B C D E

5. Cell types derived from ectoderm include ____ cells.

   1. endothelial         3. blood
   2. epidermal          4. nerve             A B C D E

6. Characteristics distinctive of the middle of the fourth week of development include:

   1. neuropores        3. branchial arches
   2. neural folds fused    4. lower limb buds      A B C D E

7. Characteristics distinctive of the fifth week of development include:

   1. eyes and nostrils     3. digital rays
   2. notches between the toes   4. eyelids         A B C D E

8. Characteristics recognizable in the embryo illustrated include:

   1. webbed fingers
   2. eyelids
   3. umbilical herniation
   4. somites

| A | B | C | D | E |
|---|---|---|---|---|
| 1,2,3 | 1,3 | 2,4 | only 4 | all correct |

9.  Events occurring during the fourth week include

    1.  appearance of limb buds      3.  closure of neuropores
    2.  formation of somites         4.  growth of neural folds      A B C D E

10. Reasonable estimates of the age of 6- to 7-week aborted
    embryos can be determined from

    1.  external characteristics
    2.  estimated time of ovulation
    3.  estimated time of fertilization
    4.  counting the number of somites                              A B C D E

11. Characteristics of embryos at the end of the 8th week of
    development include:

    1.  a large head                 3.  umbilical herniation
    2.  separate toes                4.  stubby tail                A B C D E

12. Characteristics of 5-week embryos include:

    1.  cervical sinuses             3.  foot plates
    2.  elbows                       4.  pigmented eyes             A B C D E

======================= ANSWERS, NOTES, AND EXPLANATIONS =========================

1.  D  Only 4 is correct.  Active growth and development of the neural tube into
    the primordia of the brain and spinal cord causes folding of the embryo in
    the longitudinal plane, producing head and tail folds.  The 'swinging'
    ventrally of these regions is the result of folding, not the cause of it.
    The periphery of the embryonic disc grows slowly and contributes to the
    folding process in both longitudinal and transverse planes.  Incorporation of
    the cranial part of the yolk sac into the embryo as the foregut is a result
    of folding of the head region, not a cause of it.

2.  E  All are correct.  The cranial part of the yolk sac is incorporated with
    the head fold as the foregut.  The middle part is incorporated with the
    lateral folds as the midgut, and the caudal part is incorporated with the
    tail fold as the hindgut.  The foregut, midgut, and hindgut constitute the
    primitive gut which gives rise to the epithelial lining of the digestive
    tract, except for its cranial and caudal extremities.

3.  A  1, 2, and 3 are correct.  The allantois, cloacal membrane, and primitive
    streak are carried ventrally with the tail fold.  The connecting stalk, but
    not the yolk stalk, also moves ventrally.  The yolk stalk forms in the ven-

tral region of the embryo during lateral folding.

4.  B  <u>1 and 3 are correct.</u>  The amnion, attached to the periphery of the embryonic disc, and the mass of mesoderm known as the septum transversum, are carried ventrally with the head fold.  Neither the connecting stalk nor the allantois moves with the head fold.  They are carried ventrally with the tail fold.

5.  C  <u>2 and 4 are correct.</u>  All cells of the nervous system, except microglia, are derived from ectoderm of the neural plate.  Epidermal cells of the skin are derived from surface ectoderm.  Endothelial and blood cells are derived from mesenchyme made up of angioblasts derived from mesoderm.  Microglial cells are derived from mesenchymal cells which invade the developing nervous system.

6.  A  <u>1, 2, and 3 are correct.</u>  Open neuropores, branchial arches, and fused neural folds opposite the somites are distinctive criteria for identifying embryos during the early part of the fourth week.  The limb buds do not appear until the second half of the fourth week.  Usually the upper limb buds are visible on day 26 and the lower limb buds develop about two days later.

7.  B  <u>1 and 3 are correct.</u>  Pigmented eyes, definite nostrils, and digital rays in the hand plates are characteristics of 5-week embryos.  The hand and foot plates both appear in the fifth week and are distinctive features; however, digital rays do not appear in the foot plates until early in the sixth week. Similarly, eyelids do not develop until the sixth week.

8.  A  <u>1, 2, and 3 are correct.</u>  The short, webbed fingers, the eyelids, and the early umbilical herniation are characteristics of embryos at the end of the sixth week.  The somites are not usually visible at the end of the sixth week.  Other characteristics visible in the drawing are the notches between the digital rays in the foot plates.  Herniation is usually an abnormal event, but in this case the midgut loop passes into the umbilical cord because there is no room for it in the abdomen.  This functional occurrence is often called a physiological herniation.

9.  E  <u>All are correct.</u>  These events all occur during the fourth week.  Early 4-week embryos are straight, but older embryos have a C-shaped curvature owing to longitudinal folding.  Somites are very distinctive characteristics of this week.

10.  A  <u>1, 2, and 3 are correct.</u>  External characteristics and sections of embryos give the best indications of the actual age of embryos.  Information about the estimated time of ovulation or fertilization enables one to make reasonable estimates of an embryo's age.  Hence, external characteristics of development and crown-rump measurements usually give the best indication of embryonic age.  Size alone may be an unreliable criterion because embryos may undergo slower rates of growth prior to spontaneous abortion.  After the middle of the fifth week, the number of somites is not a useful criterion for estimating embryonic age because they are indistinct.

11.  A  1, 2, and 3 are correct.  Embryos at the end of the eighth week of devel-
     opment do not have a tail.  Fan-shaped, webbed toes are characteristics of
     embryos in the seventh week, but by the end of the eighth week, all fingers
     and toes are well differentiated.  The head remains proportionately large for
     several weeks during the fetal period following the seventh week.  Intestines
     do not enter the abdomen from the cord until the tenth week of development.
     Thus the umbilical herniation is present at this time.

12.  E  All are correct.  These structures are all characteristic of 5-week
     embryos.  As the second branchial arch overgrows the third and fourth arches,
     they come to lie in a depression known as the cervical sinus.  These sinuses,
     one on each side, are usually visible externally only during the fifth week.
     Elbows and foot plates are first recognizable during the fifth week, and the
     eyes of 5-week embryos become more obvious, largely because of the develop-
     ment of retinal pigment.  Toward the end of the fifth week, the external ear
     begins to form.  The auricle develops from the fusion of six small swellings
     or hillocks that develop around the first branchial groove.

### F I V E - C H O I C E   A S S O C I A T I O N   Q U E S T I O N S

DIRECTIONS:   Each group of questions below consists of a numbered list of
descriptive words or phrases accompanied by a diagram with certain parts indicated
by letters, or by a list of lettered headings.  For each numbered word or phrase,
SELECT THE LETTERED PART OR HEADING that matches it correctly.  Then insert the
letter in the space to the right of the appropriate number.  Sometimes more than
one numbered word or phrase may be correctly matched to the same lettered part or
heading.

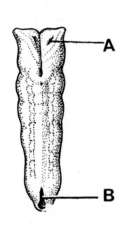

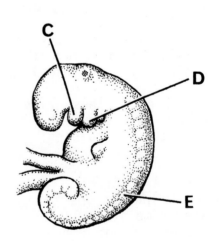

1.  __D__  Hyoid arch                4.  __C__  First branchial arch
2.  __C__  Gives rise to the mandible 5.  __B__  Neuropore
3.  __E__  Forms from paraxial mesoderm 6.  __A__  Neural fold

## ASSOCIATION QUESTIONS

A. Limb bud
B. Neuropore
C. Septum transversum
D. Cervical sinus
E. Stomodeum

7. C___ Forms major part of the diaphragm
8. B___ Primitive mouth
9. A___ Outgrowth of the body wall
10. B___ Forms as a result of the head fold
11. B___ Closes during the fourth week
12. D___ An ectodermal depression in the neck

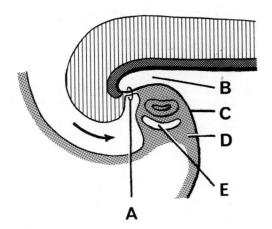

13. D___ Septum transversum
14. B___ Part of the embryonic coelom
15. A___ Oropharyngeal membrane
16. A___ Separates the amniotic cavity from the foregut
17. D___ Gives rise to the major part of the diaphragm

A. Fourth week
B. Fifth week
C. Sixth week
D. Seventh week
E. Eighth week

18. A___ Lens placodes are recognizable 4
19. C___ Umbilical herniation noticeable 6
20. B___ Retinal pigment first recognizable 8
21. A___ Lower limb buds appear 4
22. A___ Embryo essentially straight 4
23. B___ Cervical sinuses visible 5
24. E___ Tail disappears 8

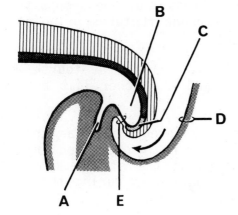

25. B___ Cloaca
26. C___ Produces embryonic mesoderm
27. B___ Separates the amniotic cavity from the hindgut
28. A___ Vestigial structure
29. D___ Amnion
30. A___ Site of blood formation in the early embryo

======================== ANSWERS, NOTES, AND EXPLANATIONS ========================

1. D  The second or hyoid branchial arch is recognizable early in the fourth week. As its name implies, this arch gives rise to the hyoid bone (part of it). Mesenchyme in this arch also gives rise to the muscles of facial expression and to various skeletal structures.

2. C  The mandibular prominences of the first pair of branchial arches give rise to the lower jaw or mandible. Rostral extensions of the first arch, called maxillary prominences, give rise to the upper jaw or maxilla.

3. E  The somites form by differentiation and division of the longitudinal columns of paraxial mesoderm into cubical segments. The somites give rise to most of the axial skeleton, the associated musculature, and the dermis of the skin.

4. C  The pointer indicates the mandibular prominence of the first branchial arch. The mandibular prominences merge with each other during the fourth week and give rise to the mandible, lower lip, and the inferior part of the face.

5. B  The caudal neuropore is indicated. Some books refer to this structure as the posterior neuropore. However, it is better to call it the caudal neuropore because it is always at the caudal end of the embryo. The neuropores (rostral and caudal) are normally closed by the end of the fourth week. The rostral neuropore closes on day 25 or 26 and the caudal neuropore usually closes about two days later. Defective closure of the caudal neuropore gives rise to a malformation called spina bifida.

6. A  The pointer indicates a neural fold in the brain region. Subsequently it fuses with the fold on the other side to form the forebrain vesicle.

7. C  The septum transversum is a mass of mesoderm that first appears cranial to the developing heart. After folding of the embryo, it lies caudal to the heart where it forms part of the primitive diaphragm. Later it develops into the central tendon of the diaphragm.

8. E  The stomodeum or primitive mouth cavity is an ectodermal depression that develops during the fourth week as the head folds. Initially it is separated from the primitive pharynx (cranial part of the foregut) by the oropharyngeal membrane. By the end of the fourth week this membrane ruptures bringing the mouth cavity into communication with the foregut.

9. A  The limb buds form on the ventrolateral body wall during the fourth week. The upper limb buds usually appear on day 25 and the lower limb buds are visible about two days later.

10. E  The stomodeum (primitive mouth cavity) and the foregut form as the head folds ventrally. The cranial part of the yolk sac is incorporated into the embryo during this longitudinal folding. At first the stomodeum and the foregut are separate cavities, but they become continuous during the fourth week when the oropharyngeal membrane ruptures.

52

11.   B  The neuropores close during the fourth week. The rostral neuropore closes on day 25 or 26 and the caudal neuropore closes about two days later. Defects of closure of the neuropores give rise to congenital malformations of the central nervous system, e.g., spina bifida.

12.   D  The cervical sinus is a depression in the surface ectoderm on each side of the future neck. It forms when the second branchial arch overgrows the third and fourth arches. The second and third arches come to lie at the bottom of a pit called the cervical sinus. It is visible externally only during the fifth week.

13.   D  The septum transversum is a mass of mesoderm that is first recognizable cranial to the pericardial coelom. After folding, it lies caudal to the heart and pericardial coelom. The septum transversum gives rise to the central tendon of the diaphragm.

14.   E  The pericardial coelom is the part of the embryonic coelom that gives rise to the pericardial cavity. It first appears in the cardiogenic mesoderm, where it lies cranial to the oropharyngeal membrane. After folding, the pericardial coelom lies ventral to the developing heart, as shown in the drawing.

15.   A  The oropharyngeal membrane develops during the third week as the prochordal plate fuses with the overlying embryonic ectoderm. This membrane ruptures during the fourth week.

16.   A  The oropharyngeal membrane separates the amniotic cavity from the foregut (primitive pharynx). Amniotic fluid may enter the primitive mouth or stomodeum, but it cannot pass into the primitive pharynx until the oropharyngeal membrane ruptures.

17.   D  The septum transversum is the first recognizable part of the developing diaphragm. It appears cranially at the end of the third week when the pericardial coelom forms. The septum transversum later forms the central tendon of the diaphragm.

18.   A  The lens placodes are recognizable during the fourth week as thickenings of the surface ectoderm. They give rise to the lens vesicles, the primordia of the lenses of the eyes.

19.   C  As the midgut loop develops, it herniates into the umbilical cord because there is not enough room for it in the abdomen. This physiological process or herniation begins during the fifth week, but the intestines do not usually form a noticeable swelling of the cord until the sixth week.

20.   B  Pigment appears in the retinae of the eyes during the fifth week, making the eyes more obvious. Eye development is first evident early in the fourth week when the optic sulci develop.

21.   A  The lower limb buds appear toward the end of the fourth week as ventrolateral swellings of the body walls. Each bud consists of a mass of mesenchyme which is covered by surface ectoderm. The upper limb buds form around the middle of the fourth week.

22.  A  The embryo is essentially straight during the early part of the fourth week.  Near the middle of the fourth week, the embryo begins to fold in the longitudinal and the horizontal planes, giving the embryo a characteristic C-shaped curvature.

23.  B  The cervical sinuses are visible externally during the fifth week.  The external openings of these sinuses usually close by the end of the fifth week.  Remnants of parts of the cervical sinuses may give rise to malformations called branchial or lateral cervical cysts.

24.  E  The tail is often visible during the early part of the eighth week, but it disappears by the end of the eighth week.

25.  B  The cloaca is the dilated caudal portion of the hindgut; the allantois enters it ventrally.  The cloaca is separated from the amniotic cavity by the cloacal membrane.

26.  C  The primitive streak appears during the early part of the third week and produces mesoderm rapidly until the end of the fourth week.  Thereafter, mesoderm production from this source slows down.

27.  E  The cloacal membrane separates the amniotic cavity from the cloacal region of the hindgut.  This membrane consists of fused layers of embryonic ectoderm and endoderm.  It is later divided into anal and urogenital membranes during the seventh week; these membranes soon rupture.

28.  A  The allantois is a rudimentary, vestigial structure that forms during the third week as a diverticulum of the caudal wall of the yolk sac.  It remains very small and gives rise to the urachus, a tubular structure that runs from the urinary bladder to the umbilicus.  Its adult derivative is the median umbilical ligament.

29.  D  The amnion forms during the second week.  It is attached to the margins of the embryonic disc and forms the wall of the amniotic sac.

30.  A  Blood begins to form in the mesenchyme around the allantois and yolk sac during the third week.  These are the only sites of blood formation until blood begins to form in the liver during the sixth week.

---

NOTES:

# THE FETAL PERIOD

The Ninth Week to Birth

## O B J E C T I V E S

BE ABLE TO:

---

o    State the significant differences between development during the
     embryonic and fetal periods, and comment on differences in the
     vulnerability of embryos and fetuses to teratogenic agents.

o    Discuss the effects of inadequate uterine environment, indicating
     the possible effects of environmental agents (e.g., viruses) and
     other factors on fetal growth and development.

o    Describe the differences between fetuses that are of low birth
     weight because of intrauterine growth retardation and those that
     are premature.

o    Write brief notes on the following techniques used for assessing
     the status of the human fetus before birth: amniocentesis,
     fetoscopy, fetal blood sampling, and ultrasonography.

---

## F I V E - C H O I C E   C O M P L E T I O N   Q U E S T I O N S

DIRECTIONS: Each of the following statements or questions is followed by five
suggested responses or completions. SELECT THE ONE BEST ANSWER in each case and
then circle the appropriate letter at the right of each question.

1.  The head constitutes almost half the fetus at the beginning of the

    A.  twelfth week            D.  stage of quickening
    B.  second trimester        E.  embryonic period
    C.  fetal period                                              A B C D E

2.  The usual measurement for estimating fetal age is

    A.  crown-rump length       D.  leg length
    B.  foot length             E.  head size
    C.  crown-heel length                                         A B C D E

<u>SELECT THE ONE BEST ANSWER</u>

3. Which of the following statements about fetal age and weight seems to be closest to the normal relationship?

    A.   8 weeks - 10  gm
    B.  12 weeks - 200 gm
    C.  20 weeks - 800 gm
    D.  26 weeks - 1000 gm
    E.  38 weeks - 4400 gm                 A B C D E

4. The fetal period begins

    A.  after all organs have completely developed
    B.  when the genitalia have distinctive characteristics
    C.  during the ninth week
    D.  at the end of the first trimester
    E.  when the developing human is viable        A B C D E

5. Sexing of fetuses is first possible from examination of the external genitalia during the _____ week.

    A.  eighth              D.  eleventh
    B.  ninth               E.  twelfth
    C.  tenth                           A B C D E

6. A fetus has a reasonable chance of surviving, if born prematurely, when its fertilization age is ____ weeks.

    A.  12                D.  20
    B.  16                E.  24
    C.  18                          A B C D E

7. Quickening, the period when fetal movements are commonly felt by the mother, usually occurs

    A.  near the end of the first trimester
    B.  around the middle of the second trimester
    C.  at the end of the second trimester
    D.  when the fetus becomes viable
    E.  during the so-called 'finishing' period     A B C D E

8. The most likely cause of very low birth weight in full-term fetuses is

    A.  maternal malnutrition
    B.  prematurity
    C.  smoking
    D.  placental insufficiency
    E.  alcoholism                      A B C D E

SELECT THE ONE BEST ANSWER

9. Amniocentesis is commonly used to

    A. diagnose the chromosomal sex of fetuses
    B. detect placental insufficiency
    C. assess the degree of erythroblastosis fetalis
    D. determine the composition of the amniotic fluid
    E. determine the age of the fetus

                       A B C D E

======================= ANSWERS, NOTES, AND EXPLANATIONS =========================

1. **C** At nine weeks, when the fetal period begins, the head constitutes almost half the fetus. Thereafter growth of the head slows down compared with the rest of the body. By the end of the twelfth week, the head represents almost one-third of the length of the fetus. The stage of quickening, or the time when the fetal movements are recognized by the mother, does not occur until the 17- to 20-week period. By this stage, the head represents a little over one-quarter of the length of the fetus.

2. **A** Crown-rump (CR) measurements are usually the most useful criteria for estimating fetal age. The length of fetuses, like infants and children, varies considerably for a given age. Crown-heel (CH) measurements are often used for older fetuses, but they are generally less useful because of the difficulty in straightening the fetus. Foot length correlates well with CR length and is particularly useful for estimating the age of incomplete or macerated fetuses. Head size is used to estimate the age of mature fetuses (e.g., after 22 weeks).

3. **D** Fetuses of about 26 weeks usually weigh about 1000 gm and survive if born prematurely. While there is no sharp limit of development, age or weight at which a fetus becomes viable, usually fetuses that are younger or weigh less do not survive. All the other weights listed are high for the ages given. For example, 8-week fetuses usually weigh about 5 gm. Full-term fetuses (38 weeks after fertilization) may weigh 4400 gm, but this is heavy. The average weight of newborn infants is 3400 gm. Heavier women usually produce heavier infants and underweight women usually have lighter infants. There is an increased frequency of low birth weights in teen-age mothers, largely because they are still growing and so have greater nutritional requirements than older women, i.e., young mothers may compete with their fetuses for nutrients.

4. **C** The fetal period begins at the beginning of the ninth week, i.e., during the first trimester. Most, but not all, organs have mainly completed their development when the fetal period begins. The external genitalia do not acquire distinctive sexual characteristics until the end of the ninth week, and their mature form is not established until the twelfth week. The intestines do not enter the abdomen until the tenth week, about one week

after the beginning of the fetal period.

5.  C  The external genitalia of male and female fetuses appear somewhat similar until the end of the twelfth week, but most people could identify the sex of 10-week embryos.  The external genitalia are fully formed by the twelfth week.

6.  E  Fetuses that weigh less than 1000 gm and are less than 24 weeks of age do not usually survive if born prematurely because of the immaturity of their respiratory systems.  By 26 to 28 weeks sufficient terminal air sacs, surfactant, and vascularity have formed for adequate gas exchange and maintenance of life.

7.  B  Fetal movements are normally felt by the mother around the middle of the second trimester of pregnancy (17 - 20 weeks).  Mothers who have been pregnant three or more times (multigravida) usually feel the fetus move sooner than mothers who are pregnant for the first time (primigravida).  The fetus begins to move before the end of the first trimester, but these movements by the relatively small fetus are too slight to be detected by the mother.

8.  D  Placental insufficiency, caused by placental defects (e.g., infarction or nonfunctional areas of the placenta) which reduce the area for passing nutrients to the embryo, produces the placental dysfunction syndrome. Impaired uterine blood flow, caused by severe hypotension and renal disease, can result in a poor passage of nutrients to the embryo.  Severe maternal malnutrition resulting from a restricted diet of poor quality may cause low birth weight, especially in teen-age mothers.  Fetuses of mothers who smoke heavily usually weigh less than fetuses of nonsmokers.  Prematurity is a common cause of low birth weight, but full-term fetuses cannot be premature.

9.  C  Withdrawal of samples of amniotic fluid (amniocentesis) is a major tool in assessing the degree of erythroblastosis fetalis (also called hemolytic disease of the fetus).  This condition results from destruction of red blood cells by maternal antibodies.  Some severely ill fetuses can be saved by giving them intrauterine blood transfusions.  Amniotic fluid is also commonly studied for detecting chromosomal abnormalities.


# M U L T I - C O M P L E T I O N   Q U E S T I O N S

DIRECTIONS:  In each of the following questions or incomplete statements ONE OR MORE of the completions is correct.  At the lower right of each question, circle A if 1, 2, and 3 are correct; B if 1 and 3 are correct; C if 2 and 4 are correct; D if only 4 is correct; and E if all are correct.


1.  Primary sources of fetal energy include:

    1.  the fetal intestines       3.  amniotic fluid
    2.  the placenta               4.  glucose                    A B C D E

| A | B | C | D | E |
|---|---|---|---|---|
| 1,2,3 | 1,3 | 2,4 | only 4 | all correct |

2. Correct statements about the fetal period include:

   1. The rate of body growth is remarkable.
   2. Changes in external body form occur rapidly.
   3. Weight gain is phenomenal during the terminal months.
   4. It is a period of rapid organ differentiation.      A B C D E

3. The fetal period is characterized by

   1. rapid growth of the body
   2. appearance of major features of external form
   3. slowdown in the growth of the head
   4. nonvulnerability to environmental agents      A B C D E

4. Factors known to affect fetal growth adversely include:

   1. impaired uteroplacental blood flow
   2. placental insufficiency
   3. severe maternal malnutrition
   4. excessive cigarette smoking      A B C D E

5. The newborn infant cannot shiver because the nervous system is not sufficiently developed, but it overcomes this by producing heat in brown fat. This fat is located chiefly

   1. in the posterior triangle     3. around the kidneys
   2. retrosternally     4. subcutaneously      A B C D E

6. Characteristics of the 9-week fetus include:

   1. intestines in umbilical cord     3. low-set ears
   2. ambiguous external genitalia     4. large head      A B C D E

7. Components of vernix caseosa include:

   1. decidual cells     3. clotted blood
   2. glandular secretions     4. epidermal cells      A B C D E

8. Usual characteristics of a viable fetus include:

   1. weighs 1000 gm or more     3. toenails
   2. red, wrinkled skin     4. eyes open      A B C D E

9. Cultured cells from amniotic fluid are used for detecting the presence or absence of

   1. inborn errors of metabolism     3. 21 trisomy
   2. sex chromosome abnormalities     4. twins      A B C D E

| A | B | C | D | E |
|---|---|---|---|---|
| 1,2,3 | 1,3 | 2,4 | only 4 | all correct |

10. Prior to 22 weeks, a normal fetus born prematurely dies because its

    1. brown fat has not formed
    ②. nervous system is not sufficiently well developed
    3. cardiovascular system is immature
    ④. lungs are not sufficiently well developed                    A B C D E

======================= ANSWERS, NOTES, AND EXPLANATIONS =========================

1. C  2 and 4 are correct.  Glucose is the primary source of energy for fetal metabolism.  The insulin required for the metabolism of glucose is secreted by the fetal pancreas.  Glucose in the maternal blood also crosses the placenta quickly and enters the fetal blood.  The placenta also synthesizes glycogen during early pregnancy from maternal glucose, and releases glucose into the fetus by glycogenolysis.

2. B  1 and 3 are correct.  Changes in external body form take place quite slowly through slight differences in the relative growth rates of the various parts of the body.  Although much differentiation of tissues and organs occurs during the fetal period, the changes produced take place over several months.  In some cases (e.g., the brain and adrenal glands), the differentiation continues for several years after birth.

3. B  1 and 3 are correct.  Two main characteristics of the fetal period are rapid growth of the body with a relative slowdown in the growth of the head.  All major features of external form appear during the embryonic period.  Although the fetus is far less vulnerable to teratogens than the embryo, the final development of certain structures can be deranged, e.g, the brain and external genitalia.  Certain viruses (rubella virus and cytomegalovirus) are particularly harmful to the brain and eyes during the fetal period.

4. E  All are correct.  Placental insufficiency results from placental defects (e.g., an infarction, i.e., an area of coagulation necrosis in the placenta) that result in areas of the placenta becoming non-functional in the transfer of nutrients to the fetus.  It is often difficult to separate the effects of these changes from the effects of reduced maternal blood flow to the placenta.  Impaired uteroplacental blood flow can result from severe hypotension or renal disease.  Severe maternal malnutrition or excessive cigarette smoking, or both, can also cause retarded fetal growth, but their effects are not usually so profound as those resulting from placental insufficiency.

5. A  1, 2, and 3 are correct.  White fat is deposited subcutaneously, especially during the last six to eight weeks of gestation.  Brown fat is deposited

60

mainly during the 17 - 20 week period. It appears brown because it has a very rich capillary supply, and its cells are rich in cytochromes that contain a colored component. Brown adipose tissue plays an important role in regulating body temperature in the newborn. It produces heat by oxidizing fatty acids.

6. E  <u>All are correct</u>.  Intestines in the umbilical cord and a large head are distinctive characteristics. The intestines return to the abdomen during the tenth week. The external ears gradually move cranially to their usual position as the jaws develop, but do not reach their final position until the middle of the second trimester. Female fetuses at this stage can be wrongly diagnosed as males because the clitoris is relatively large.

7. C  <u>2 and 4 are correct</u>.  Vernix caseosa is a greasy, cheese-like substance that covers the skin of older fetuses. It consists of a mixture of a fatty secretion from the sebaceous glands and dead epidermal cells. Vernix caseosa is thought to protect the fetus's skin from abrasions, chapping, and hardening as a result of being bathed in the amniotic fluid.

8. B  <u>1 and 3 are correct</u>.  While there are no definite signs of viability, usually fetuses that weigh 1000 gm or more and are 26 or more weeks old, have a reasonable chance of survival. The toenails are formed by 30 weeks when the chances for survival are fairly good. If the skin is red and wrinkled, the fetus is usually less than 26 weeks, or has suffered intrauterine growth retardation. In these cases, very little white fat forms and brown fat is reduced or absent. While it is true that the eyes are usually open in viable fetuses, the eyes of very young fetuses (e.g., 9 weeks) are also open.

9. A  <u>1, 2, and 3 are correct</u>.  Fetal sex can also be detected by examining the sex chromosome complement of the cells, but sex chromatin studies of uncultured cells may be used for this purpose. Detection of chromosomal abnormalities that will result in severe physical and mental abnormalities is a common reason for studying cultured amniotic cells. These studies permit prenatal diagnosis of severe diseases for which there is no effective treatment.

10. C  <u>2 and 4 are correct</u>.  The lungs do not have sufficient capillary networks or terminal air sacs to permit maintenance of life. Prior to 22 weeks the pulmonary vascular bed is unable to accommodate the entire cardiac output, so respiratory difficulties develop. During the 26- to 28-week period, the nervous system matures to the point where it can control rhythmic breathing. Brown fat forms in previable fetuses and the cardiovascular system is completely formed by the beginning of the fetal period.

# F I V E - C H O I C E   A S S O C I A T I O N   Q U E S T I O N S

DIRECTIONS: Each group of questions below consists of a numbered list of descriptive words or phrases accompanied by a diagram with certain parts indicated by letters, or by a list of lettered headings. For each numbered word or phrase, SELECT THE LETTERED PART OR HEADING that matches it correctly. Then insert the letter in the space to the right of the appropriate number. Sometimes more than one numbered word or phrase may be correctly matched to the same lettered part or heading.

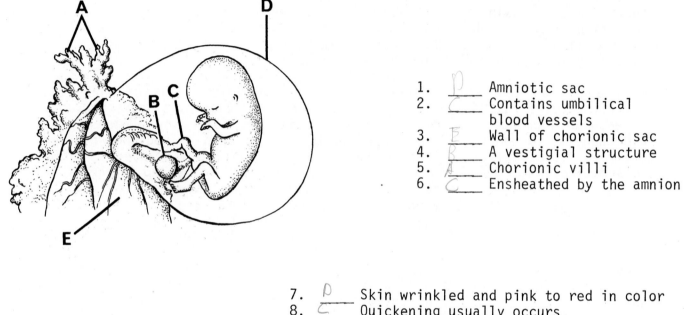

1. _D_ Amniotic sac
2. _C_ Contains umbilical blood vessels
3. _E_ Wall of chorionic sac
4. _B_ A vestigial structure
5. _A_ Chorionic villi
6. _C_ Ensheathed by the amnion

7. _D_ Skin wrinkled and pink to red in color
8. _C_ Quickening usually occurs
9. _B_ Skeleton first shows clearly on x-ray films
10. _A_ Sex becomes distinguishable externally
11. _C_ Eyebrows, head hair and lanugo hair first visible
12. _A_ The head constitutes half the fetus
13. _E_ The fetus has good chance of surviving if born prematurely
14. _C_ Brown fat begins to form
15. _A_ Stage of initial activity of fetus

A. 8 to 12 weeks
B. 13 to 16 weeks
C. 17 to 20 weeks
D. 21 to 25 weeks
E. 26 to 29 weeks

======================== ANSWERS, NOTES, AND EXPLANATIONS ========================

1. D The amniotic sac contains amniotic fluid which permits free movement of the fetus and permits symmetrical external growth. This fluid also cushions

the fetus against jolts the mother may receive, and helps to control the fetus's body temperature.

2.  C  The umbilical cord contains the umbilical vessels, normally two arteries and one vein.  The vein carries nutrients and oxygenated blood to the fetus and the arteries carry deoxgenated blood and waste products to the placenta where the carbon dioxide and waste substances are transferred to the maternal blood for disposal.

3.  E  The chorionic sac at this stage is normally embedded in the endometrium and contains the embryo in its amniotic sac.  Chorionic villi cover most of the outer wall of the sac at this stage.  Some villi have degenerated because they were compressed and received insufficient blood supply for survival.

4.  B  The remnant of the primitive yolk sac indicated is a vestigial structure, serving no function at this stage.  Part of the early yolk sac was incorporated into the embryo during the fourth week as the primitive gut. Within a few weeks, the remnant of the yolk sac indicated will degenerate and disappear.

5.  A  The chorionic villi project from the wall of the chorionic sac.  These very important parts of the placenta are normally embedded in the endometrium and bathed in maternal blood.  It is through the villi that the exchange of nutrients between the mother and fetus takes place.

6.  C  The umbilical cord has an external investment or covering of amnion.  As the amniotic sac enlarges, the amnion gradually forms the outer covering of the cord.

7.  D  During the 21- to 25-week period, the skin is usually wrinkled and pink to red in color because blood in the capillaries has become visible through the thin, transparent skin.  During the subsequent four weeks, considerable subcutaneous fat forms, smoothing out many of the wrinkles.

8.  C  During the 17- to 20-week period, movements of the fetus are usually felt by the mother for the first time; this event is known as quickening. Although the fetus begins to move several weeks earlier, these movements are too slight to be felt by the mother.

9.  B  Towards the end of the 13- to 16-week period, the skeleton shows clearly on x-ray films.  Roentgenography (photography by means of x- or roentgen rays) may be used to detect multiple births or maternal pelvic abnormalities. Care is taken to prevent the fetus from receiving too much radiation because of the possible adverse effects on its germ cells and developing brain.

10.  A  Sex first becomes distinguishable during the 8- to 12-week period.  At 8 weeks, the external genitalia of males and females appear similar.  By the end of the ninth week, it is usually possible to differentiate between males and females, but the mature form of the genitalia is not reached until the twelfth week.

11. C The 17- to 20-week period is important for several reasons. Fetal movements are first felt by the mother; vernix caseosa forms and affords protection for the fetal skin; body hair (lanugo), head hair and the eyebrows become visible, and brown fat begins to form. This specialized fat is an important site of heat production.

12. A At the beginning of the fetal period, the head constitutes about half the length of the fetus. Thereafter there is a relative slowdown in the growth of the head compared to the rest of the body. The large head in early fetuses results from the very rapid development of the brain during the embryonic period.

13. E By the 26- to 29-week period, the fetus has a reasonably good chance of surviving if it is born prematurely, but the mortality rate is usually high because of respiratory difficulties. The fetus is able to survive primarily because its respiratory and nervous systems have matured to the stage where rhythmic breathing can occur. Capillary proliferation in the lungs becomes very active during this period. Prior to the 26- to 28-week period, the pulmonary vascular bed is unable to accommodate the entire cardiac output and so gas exchange in the lungs may not be adequate to support life.

14. C Brown fat begins to form during the 17- to 20-week period. Heat is produced in this specialized adipose tissue, particularly during the newborn period, by oxidizing fatty acids. Brown fat is found chiefly on the floor of the posterior triangle of the neck, posterior to the sternum, and in the perirenal regions.

15. A The stage of initial activity is during the 8- to 12-week period. By the end of 12 weeks, stroking the lips of a fetus will cause it to begin sucking, and if the eyelids are stroked there is a reflex response. These early movements of the fetus are too slight to be felt by the mother. She cannot usually detect fetal movements until the 17- to 20-week period; these movements, called quickening, constitute a positive sign of a living fetus.

---

NOTES:

# THE PLACENTA AND FETAL MEMBRANES

## O B J E C T I V E S

BE ABLE TO:

_____

o   Construct and label simple drawings showing the following fetal
    membranes: amnion, chorion, yolk sac, and allantois.  Discuss the
    fate of each of the above fetal membranes.

o   Describe the development of the placenta, using drawings to show
    the essential features of placental structure and function.

o   Illustrate the placental membrane (placental barrier) and discuss
    the transfer of materials between the fetal and maternal blood
    streams.

o   List the main activities of the placenta, discussing their role
    in maintaining pregnancy and in promoting embryonic development.

o   Construct and label simple drawings showing the gross and
    microscopic structure of the placenta and umbilical cord after
    birth.

o   Illustrate with sketches and discuss the embryological basis of
    multiple births, with special emphasis on twinning.

_____

## F I V E - C H O I C E   C O M P L E T I O N   Q U E S T I O N S

DIRECTIONS:  Each of the following statements or questions is followed by five
suggested responses or completions. SELECT THE ONE BEST ANSWER in each case and
then circle the appropriate letter at the right of each question.

1.   Primary chorionic villi are recognizable by the end of the
     _____ week.

     A. first            D. fourth
     B. second           E. fifth
     C. third                                           A B C D E

2.   The most distinctive characteristic of a primary chorionic
     villus is its

     A. outer syncytial layer        D. cytotrophoblastic core
     B. cytotrophoblastic shell      E. villous appearance
     C. mesenchymal core                                A B C D E

SELECT THE ONE BEST ANSWER

3.  Villi are designated as secondary chorionic villi
    when they

    A.  contact the decidua basalis
    B.  are covered by syncytiotrophoblast
    C.  develop a mesenchymal core
    D.  have branch villi
    E.  have capillaries                                    A B C D E

4.  When villi are vascularized, they are best called ____ villi.

    A.  branch                      D.  anchoring
    B.  stem                        E.  true
    C.  tertiary                                            A B C D E

5.  The most important region of the decidua for nutrition of
    the embryo is the decidua ____ .

    A.  vera                        D.  basalis
    B.  capsularis                  E.  none of the above
    C.  parietalis                                          A B C D E

6.  Which of the following regions of the decidua degenerates
    and disappears during the second trimester of pregnancy?

    A.  Decidua vera                D.  Decidua basalis
    B.  Decidua capsularis          E.  None of the above
    C.  Decidua parietalis                                  A B C D E

7.  Contents of the intervillous space normally include each
    of the following substances, except:

    A.  oxygen                      D.  fetal blood
    B.  carbon dioxide              E.  electrolytes
    C.  maternal blood                                      A B C D E

8.  Which of the following materials usually do not cross the
    placental membrane (barrier)?

    A.  Free fatty acids            D.  Vitamins
    B.  Steroid hormones            E.  Drugs
    C.  Bacteria                                            A B C D E

9.  The substance exchanged most rapidly and freely between the
    mother and her embryo is

    A.  water                       D.  free fatty acids
    B.  vitamins                    E.  minerals
    C.  antibodies                                          A B C D E

SELECT THE ONE BEST ANSWER

10. The most characteristic feature of the maternal surface of the placenta is its

    A. attachment of the cord      D. shreds of decidua
    B. amniotic covering          E. intervillous spaces
    C. cotyledons                                 A B C D E

11. At which of the following stages of development is division of embryonic material not likely to result in normal monozygotic twinning?

    A. Two-cell stage         D. Primitive streak
    B. Morula                 E. Bilaminar embryo
    C. Blastocyst                                A B C D E

12. An examination of the placenta and fetal membranes of male twins revealed two amnions, two chorions, and fused placentas. Twinning most likely resulted from

    A. dispermy
    B. fertilization of two ova
    C. superfecundation
    D. fertilization of one ovum
    E. the effect of gonadotropins                     A B C D E

======================= ANSWERS, NOTES, AND EXPLANATIONS =========================

1. B  The appearance of primary chorionic villi is a distinctive feature of the second week of human development. Commencing on about day nine and continuing until the fourth week, there is intense growth and differentiation of the chorion.

2. D  Early in the second week, irregular processes of syncytiotrophoblast form; outgrowths of cytotrophoblast soon extend into these syncytiotrophoblast processes. When these primordial villous structures acquire cores of cytotrophoblast, they are called primary chorionic villi. They represent the first stage in the development of the histological structure of the chorionic villi of the mature placenta.

3. C  The distinctive histological characteristic of a secondary chorionic villus is its loose core of mesenchyme. This embryonic connective tissue is derived from the extraembryonic somatic mesoderm. This change occurs at the end of the second week, or early in the third week of development.

4. C  The final stage in the elaboration of the histological structure of chorionic villi results in the formation of tertiary villi. The adjective 'true'

is sometimes used to describe villi in the final stage of development, but tertiary is the better term and is the internationally accepted one. If the term true villus is used, it is implied that there are false villi. The arterio-capillary-venous system within the core of each villus develops by the end of the third week, and these vessels become connected with those in the chorion, connecting stalk (future umbilical cord), and embryo. Thus, by the end of the third week a simple circulatory system is established.

5. D The gravid (pregnant) endometrium underlying the conceptus, called the decidua basalis, constitutes the maternal part of the placenta. The placenta is primarily an organ for the interchange of material between the maternal and fetal blood streams, e.g., oxygen, carbon dioxide, and food materials.

6. B As the conceptus enlarges, the decidua capsularis bulges into the uterine cavity and becomes greatly attenuated. Eventually it fuses with the decidua parietalis, obliterating the uterine cavity. By about 22 weeks, reduced blood supply to the decidua capsularis results in its degeneration and subsequent disappearance. Although the epithelium of the decidua parietalis eventually disappears, its other layers persist.

7. D There is normally no intermingling of the fetal and maternal blood streams. However, there is evidence that some fetal and maternal red blood cells cross the placental membrane. The circulation of maternal blood in the intervillous space is of particular importance in the supply of oxygen, electrolytes, and nutrient substances to the fetus, and for the removal of its waste products (e.g., carbon dioxide and urea).

8. C It is generally believed that bacteria are not transferred across the placenta. However, it is important to realize that other microorganisms (e.g., rubella virus, cytomegalovirus, and Toxoplasma gondii) do cross the placenta and may cause congenital malformations. When present in the maternal blood, bacteria may form the origin of an infection which subsequently may rupture into the fetal placental circulation. In general, almost all substances are probably able to cross the placenta to some extent. It is the rate and the mechanism of crossing which differ. The old sieve-like concept of the placenta has been replaced by a more complex view, in which the placenta selectively controls the rates of transfer of a wide variety of materials.

9. A Water is readily transferred between the mother and the embryo/fetus, and in increasing amounts as pregnancy progresses, but the factors governing the net transfer of water are multiple and complex. Each solute transferred to the embryo and utilized, liberates water molecules. Also the oxidation of glucose and other nutrients results in the production of water molecules.

10. C The 15 to 30 cotyledons give the maternal surface of the placenta a characteristic cobblestone appearance. They are separated by grooves formerly occupied by the placental septa. Though shreds of the decidua basalis are attached to the surface of the cotyledons, they are clearly identifiable only under the microscope. The attachment of the umbilical cord and the amniotic covering are features of the fetal surface of the placenta.

11. D  After the end of the second week and establishment of a primitive streak, it is unlikely that separate monozygotic twins can develop. If partitioning of the embryonic disc during the second week is incomplete, conjoined twins will result. Studies of the chorions, amnions, and placentas of monozygotic twins indicate that most partitioning of embryonic formative material occurs during the blastocyst stage, between 4 and 7 days. Separation of the inner cell mass into two parts results in the formation of two embryonic discs, two primitive streaks, and separate embryos.

12. B  Usually the presence of two chorionic sacs indicates dizygotic ('unlike' or 'fraternal') twinning. From two-thirds to three-quarters of all human twins are dizygotic. The placentas and membranes observed could be associated with monozygotic twinning because in 25 to 30 percent of cases, monozygotic twinning results from separation of the first two or more blastomeres. This results in the formation of two amniotic sacs and two chorionic sacs, and separate or fused placentas. Thus, it may be difficult to determine if twins with the kind of membranes described are monozygotic or dizygotic. If they are of opposite sex or have different blood types, they are obviously dizygotic. Like-sex twins, as in this case, may be considered monozygotic when they have the same blood type and strongly resemble each other in such characteristics as hair and eye color, fingerprints, and shape of the external ear.

## M U L T I - C O M P L E T I O N   Q U E S T I O N S

DIRECTIONS:  In each of the following questions or incomplete statements ONE OR MORE of the completions is correct. At the lower right of each question, circle A if 1, 2, and 3 are correct; B if 1 and 3 are correct; C if 2 and 4 are correct; D if only 4 is correct; and E if all are correct.

1.  During the first two weeks of development, which of the following may have a role in the early nutrition of the embryo?

   1.  Maternal blood          3.  Decidual cells
   2.  Yolk sac                4.  Uterine glands          A B C D E

2.  The placenta performs which of the following functional activities?

   1.  Excretion               3.  Endocrine secretion
   2.  Nutrition               4.  Gas exchange             A B C D E

3.  Amniotic fluid is concerned in which of the following functional activities?

   1.  Protection
   2.  Fluid exchange
   3.  Temperature regulation
   4.  Gas exchange                                        A B C D E

69

| A | B | C | D | E |
|---|---|---|---|---|
| 1,2,3 | 1,3 | 2,4 | only 4 | all correct |

4. Contributions to the amniotic fluid come from the

   1. fetal lungs
   2. maternal blood
   3. fetal kidneys
   4. amniotic cells

   A B C D E

5. The decidua basalis

   1. lies between the villous chorion and the myometrium
   2. forms the 'roof' of the placenta
   3. supplies blood to the intervillous spaces
   4. is composed of tissues of fetal origin

   A B C D E

6. The placental membrane

   1. becomes relatively thicker as pregnancy advances
   2. is interposed between the fetal and maternal blood
   3. initially consists of three layers of tissue
   4. is composed entirely of tissues of fetal origin

   A B C D E

7. Mechanisms involved in placental transfer of material include:

   1. facilitated diffusion
   2. pinocytosis
   3. active transport
   4. simple diffusion

   A B C D E

8. Hormones synthesized by the syncytiotrophoblast include:

   1. Gonadotropin (hCG)
   2. Progesterone
   3. Somatomammotropin (hCS)
   4. Estrogens

   A B C D E

9. The allantois is involved in formation of the

   1. umbilical cord
   2. urachus
   3. blood cells
   4. primordial germ cells

   A B C D E

10. Human twins may be considered monozygotic if they

    1. exhibit mirror-imaging
    2. have identical blood groups
    3. share a chorionic sac
    4. are of the same sex

    A B C D E

11. At which stage(s) of development may separation of embryonic material occur and usually give rise to separate monozygotic twins?

    1. Two-cell stage
    2. Morula
    3. 5-day blastocyst
    4. 10-day blastocyst

    A B C D E

| A | B | C | D | E |
|-----|-----|-----|--------|-------------|
| 1,2,3 | 1,3 | 2,4 | only 4 | all correct |

12. Correct statements about the umbilical cord include:

    1. It usually attaches near the center of the placenta.
    2. It may not be attached to the placenta.
    3. It normally contains two arteries and one vein.
    4. False knots may be hazardous to the fetus.       A B C D E

======================= ANSWERS, NOTES, AND EXPLANATIONS =========================

1. E  **All are correct.** During the first week, embryonic cells augment their meager supply of nutrients by obtaining material from secretions of the uterine tube and the uterus. These substances diffuse through the zona pellucida. When the morula enters the uterus, the uterine glands are actively secreting a mixture (sometimes called 'uterine milk') of protein, mucopolysaccharide, glycogen and lipid. The developing embryonic cells also obtain their oxygen from the uterine secretions. During the second week, the embryo derives its nourishment mainly from maternal blood in the lacunar networks. As implantation occurs, uterine glands and capillaries are destroyed; thus, the fluid surrounding the blastocyst consists of extravasated (escaped) blood, uterine glandular contents, and other cell products. The large decidual cells are filled with glycogen and lipid, and undoubtedly these materials enter the maternal blood as these cells are destroyed. The nutritive fluid around the chorionic sac of the embryo is called embryotroph or histiotrophy; embryotroph is a much better term as it indicates that the fluid is a source of nutrition (Greek trophe means nutrition) for the embryo. This fluid diffuses through the trophoblast into the blastocyst cavity. The yolk sac is undoubtably concerned in the transfer of nutritive fluid to the embryo from the trophoblast and extraembryonic coelom during the second week. The fact that blood vessels first appear on the yolk sac supports the view that it has an active role in the nutrition of the embryo.

2. E  **All are correct.** The basic functional activity of the placenta is to bring the maternal and fetal circulations into close proximity to permit the exchange of materials (oxygen, carbon dioxide, nutrients, waste products, etc). It also secretes hormones and synthesizes glycogen, cholesterol, and fatty acids. Thus, the placenta is a unique organ because it can perform the activities of a lung, a digestive organ, the liver, a kidney, and an endocrine gland.

3. A  **1,2, and 3 are correct.** Amniotic fluid is not involved in gas exchange. It protects the embryo by cushioning it against jolts the mother may receive. It also prevents adhesion of the amnion to the embryo as may occur with oligohydramnios (small amount of amniotic fluid). There is a rapid exchange of water molecules between the maternal circulation, the fetal circulation, and

71

the amniotic fluid. The fetal kidneys and intestine, and probably the amniochorionic membrane, are involved in this exchange. Amniotic fluid is believed to have an important role in temperature regulation of the embryo.

4. E  All are correct.  Initially amniotic fluid appears to be produced by the amniotic cells, either by filtration or secretion. Some fluid also comes from secretions of the mucous cells of the tracheobronchial tree (estimated to be as much as 30 ml per day near term). Fluid from the maternal blood is believed to be the major source of amniotic fluid, especially during the embryonic period. It probably passes through the amniochorionic membrane adjacent to the decidua parietalis and at the fetal surface of the placenta. When the fetal kidneys begin to function, fetal urine is added to the amniotic fluid (about a half-liter daily by full term).

5. B  1 and 3 are correct.  The decidua basalis is the part of the gravid endometrium underlying the conceptus and forming the maternal part of the placenta. Thus it lies between the villous chorion (fetal part of the placenta) and the muscle layer (myometrium) of the uterus. Up to 100 spiral arteries in the decidua basalis open into the intervillous space. Maternal blood is propelled from these arteries in jet-like fountains by the maternal blood pressure. The decidua basalis is composed entirely of maternal tissues.

6. C  2 and 4 are correct.  The tissues across which transport of material occurs are known collectively as the placental membrane (barrier). It is a composite membrane consisting of four main layers during early pregnancy: two layers of trophoblast (syncytiotrophoblast and cytotrophoblast); stroma (mesenchyme) in the villi; and the endothelium of the fetal capillary. In addition, material must pass through the basement membrane of the trophoblast and of the fetal capillary or sinusoid. After about 20 weeks, the placental membrane becomes greatly thinned and the stroma much reduced. The cytotrophoblast usually disappears, the number of capillaries greatly increases, and the surface area of the placenta becomes greater.

7. E  All are correct.  Simple diffusion is a process of movement of substances (e.g., oxygen, carbon dioxide, low molecular weight substances including electrolytes and drugs) across the placental membrane from an area of high concentration to one of lower concentration. Transfer ceases when equilibrium is reached. Facilitated diffusion also depends on a concentration gradient, but there is a carrier mechanism in addition which permits more rapid and specific transfer of material (e.g., glucose transport appears to be by this mechanism). Active transport involves transfer against a gradient and is an energy-using metabolic process. Transport of essential amino acids and water-soluable vitamins occurs by this mechanism. Pinocytosis, engulfment of particles and droplets by the trophoblast, is not believed to be of much significance in the transfer of nutrients, but the process is important from an immunological standpoint. The transport of globulins, lipoproteins, phospholipids, and other molecules too large for diffusion appears to be by this mechanism.

8. E  All are correct.  It is well established that the placenta produces the two protein hormones listed (hCG and hCS or hPL). Current opinion is that chorionic thyrotropin and corticotropin are also formed by the placenta.

Estrogens and progesterones are the main steroids known to be produced by the placenta. When the placenta begins to produce large amounts of progesterone, the corpus luteum of pregnancy slowly begins to retrogress (degenerate); usually this begins at about 20 weeks.

9. A **1, 2, and 3 are correct**. The allantois (from Greek _allantos_ meaning 'sausage') develops during the third week as a diverticulum of the yolk sac, and grows for a short distance into the umbilical cord. The allantoic blood vessels around it become the umbilical blood vessels. Thus, the allantois contributes to the formation of the umbilical cord. The allantois can be identified, between the umbilical arteries, in transverse sections through the proximal end of the umbilical cord until about the end of the first trimester. Cells formed in the wall of the yolk sac and allantois are the sole source of blood cells, until hemopoiesis begins in the fetal liver at about six weeks. The intraembryonic portion of the allantois becomes a thick tube, the urachus, which runs between the umbilicus and the urinary bladder. Usually the urachus becomes the median umbilical ligament after birth, but it may give rise to various urachal malformations. Primordial germ cells have been observed on the yolk sac near the origin of the allantois, but not on the wall of the allantois.

10. A **1, 2, and 3 are correct**. Dizygotic (DZ) twins may be of the same sex, but they never share a chorionic sac. The only kind of placenta which is diagnostic of monozygotic (MZ) twinning is the monochorionic type. Separate placentas and membranes (amnions and chorions), and fused placentas with separate amniotic sacs can be observed in both types of twins. Often some placental vessels of MZ twins join; however, these anastomoses are usually well balanced so that neither twin suffers. If one twin receives a disproportionate share of blood, fetal transfusion results in which there is a wide discrepancy in the size of the twins. In about one-quarter of MZ twins, the phenomenon of lateral inversion or mirror-imaging is present, e.g., hair whorls or dental anomalies are on opposite sides in the twins. Thus, if present, mirror-imaging is diagnostic of MZ twinning.

11. E **All are correct**. About 75 percent of monozygotic (MZ) twins share a single placenta and chorionic sac, but have separate amniotic sacs. This results from duplication of the inner cell mass between days 4 and 7. The separation of the inner cell mass into two parts gives rise to two amniotic sacs and two embryonic discs within the same chorionic sac. About 25 percent of monozygotic twins have separate, but secondarily fused placentas and chorions. Both MZ and DZ twins can have fused placentas and membranes; separation of the early blastomeres (2-cell stage to morula) would give rise to this situation. Division of the embryonic disc on days 8 to 13 occurs uncommonly, but this process always gives rise to one placenta, one chorionic sac, and one amniotic sac. If division is incomplete, a variety of conjoined twins results. It is very doubtful that twinning can occur after the end of the second week because the development of a primitive streak initiates the development of a single embryo.

12. A **1, 2, and 3 are correct** False knots, as the term implies, are not knots; they represent loops in the umbilical vessels and are of no significance.

However, a true knot may be hazardous to the fetus if it tightens enough to obstruct blood flow in the cord. Uncommonly, the umbilical vessels run between the amnion and chorion before entering the placenta. This condition is called a velamentous insertion of the cord. In about one percent of cords, only one artery is present; this condition may be associated with congenital malformations, particularly of the cardiovascular system.

## F I V E - C H O I C E   A S S O C I A T I O N   Q U E S T I O N S

DIRECTIONS: Each group of questions below consists of a numbered list of descriptive words or phrases accompanied by a diagram with certain parts indicated by letters, or by a list of lettered headings. For each numbered word or phrase, SELECT THE LETTERED PART OR HEADING that matches it correctly. Then insert the letter in the space to the right of the appropriate number. Sometimes more than one numbered word or phrase may be correctly matched to the same lettered part or heading.

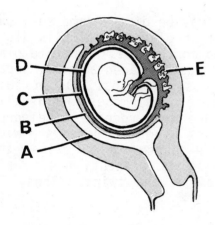

1. _B_  Decidua capsularis
2. _D_  Ensheaths the umbilical cord
3. _C_  Smooth chorion
4. _A_  Decidua parietalis
5. _B_  Fuses with the decidua parietalis
6. _B_  Maternal part of the placenta

A. Separate placentas and membranes
B. Fibrinoid
C. Amniochorionic membrane
D. Monochorionic placenta
E. Syncytial knot

7. _D_  Occurs only in monozygotic twins
8. _E_  Nuclear aggregation
9. _A_  Unusual in monozygotic twins
10. _B_  Stains intensely with eosin
11. _C_  Extends into the cervix during labor
12. _B_  Forms on the surfaces of chorionic villi

ASSOCIATION QUESTIONS

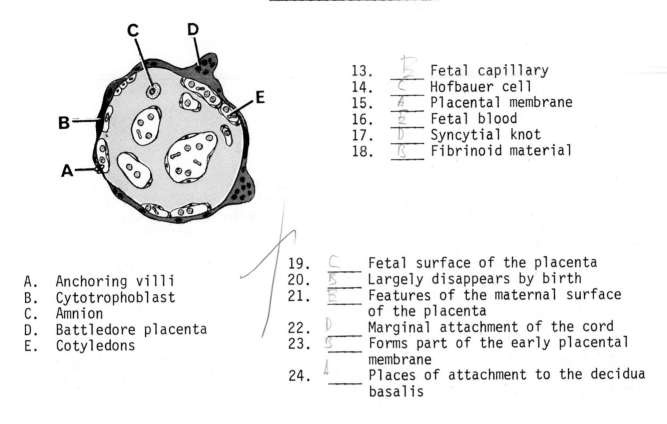

13. _B_ Fetal capillary
14. _C_ Hofbauer cell
15. _A_ Placental membrane
16. _E_ Fetal blood
17. _D_ Syncytial knot
18. _B_ Fibrinoid material

A. Anchoring villi
B. Cytotrophoblast
C. Amnion
D. Battledore placenta
E. Cotyledons

19. _C_ Fetal surface of the placenta
20. _B_ Largely disappears by birth
21. _E_ Features of the maternal surface of the placenta
22. _D_ Marginal attachment of the cord
23. _B_ Forms part of the early placental membrane
24. _A_ Places of attachment to the decidua basalis

========================= ANSWERS, NOTES, AND EXPLANATIONS =========================

1.  B   The decidua capsularis is the part of the decidua (gravid endometrium) that encapsulates the luminal surface of the implanted conceptus.  At the stage illustrated, it is fused with the smooth chorion.  Together the amnion and chorion form the amniochorionic membrane.

2.  D   As the amniotic sac enlarges, it gradually obliterates the chorionic cavity and ensheaths the umbilical cord.  The amnion becomes the epithelial covering of the cord.

3.  C   The chorion laeve or smooth chorion is continuous with the chorionic plate ('roof') of the placenta.  From the third to eighth week, the region of the chorionic sac indicated, was covered by villi.  The villi degenerated as the amniotic sac enlarged and pressed the chorion against the decidua capsularis.  This reduced the  blood supply to the villi and resulted in their degeneration.

4.  A   The decidua parietalis refers to the endometrium lining parts of the uterus not directly involved with the conceptus, i.e., endometrium not designated as decidua capsularis or decidua basalis.

75

5.  B  The decidua capsularis enlarges with the growing conceptus and bulges into the uterine cavity. Eventually the decidua capsularis fuses with the decidua parietalis, thus obliterating the uterine cavity. By about 22 weeks, reduced blood supply to the attenuated decidua capsularis causes it to degenerate and gradually disappear.

6.  E  The decidua basalis forms the maternal part of the placenta. The fetal part is formed by the villous chorion (chorion frondosum). Together they form a unique fetomaternal organ, the placenta, the basic function of which is to bring the maternal and fetal circulations into close proximity in order to permit effective exchange of materials.

7.  D  A monochorionic twin placenta, associated with twins in separate amniotic sacs, occurs only with monozygotic twins; thus this type of placenta is diagnostic of monozygotic twinning. Often the twins have a common fetal placental circulation which can be demonstrated by injecting colored latex into the vessels of one of the umbilical cords. The latex soon appears in the vessels on the other twin's side of the placenta. This placental condition may produce circulatory imbalance resulting in diminished blood supply to one of the twins, the so-called transfusion syndrome. With a marked degree of imbalance, considerable differences in the development of the fetuses may occur.

8.  E  At some sites, the placental membrane (syncytiotrophoblast) of mature placentas shows protuberances or sprouts of cytoplasm containing aggregations of syncytiotrophoblastic nuclei, called syncytial knots. Some knots break off and float in the intervillous space. They may pass into the maternal circulation through the uterine veins, and lodge in the capillaries of the lung. This occurrence is not considered to be of clinical significance because these nuclear masses are believed to degenerate and disappear.

9.  A  Monozygotic twins that develop following separation of the early blastomeres have separate placentas and membranes. Because the early blastocysts are enclosed in the same zona pellucida, they usually implant close together and their chorionic sacs and placentas usually fuse. This arrangement of the placentas and membranes commonly occurs with dizygotic twins. Thus other criteria must be used to determine what type of twins was born, e.g., comparison of genetic markers such as blood groups or serum factors. A difference in any genetic marker indicates dizygosity. Similarities in several genetic markers does not prove monozygosity because any two children of the same parents might resemble each other in these genetic markers by chance. Many other genetic markers must then be studied before monozygosity is proved or highly probable.

10. B  Fibrinoid stains intensely with eosin in hematoxylin and eosin-stained sections of villi. It has been shown to be a mucoprotein-mucopolysaccharide complex. It is present in younger placentas, but becomes increasingly abundant in older placentas. It appears at the junction between fetal and maternal tissues, in the chorionic plate (roof of the placenta), and on the surfaces of villi. Fibrinoid is believed to be important in the prevention of rejection of the placenta and fetus by the mother. These age changes in the fibrinoid are closely linked with the functional efficiency of the

placenta, because this amorphous material reduces the surface area of the placental membrane (fetomaternal barrier) available for exchange of materials.

11. C  The chorion, to which the amnion is fused, extends into the cervical canal during the first stage of labor and helps to dilate the cervix. When the fused layers of amnion and chorion (the amniochorionic membrane) rupture, the amniotic fluid escapes through the cervix and vagina.

12. B  Fibrinoid is an eosinophilic, homogeneous substance that forms on the surfaces of villi and reduces the area of tissues through which exchange of materials between the maternal and fetal circulations may take place. It consists of fibrin and other unidentified substances.

13. E  The fetal capillaries, embedded in the stroma of the chorionic villi, are part of an arterio-capillary-venous system carrying the fetal blood. As pregnancy advances, the capillaries increase in size and their walls eventually come into intimate relation with the syncytiotrophoblast. The endothelium of the capillary is separated from the syncytiotrophoblast by only an extremely delicate network of reticular fibers.

14. C  Hofbauer cells are large cells in the mesenchymal core of chorionic villi. The vacuoles in these cells contain mucopolysaccharides, mucoproteins, and lipids. Although the complete role of these cells is not understood, it is generally believed that they are macrophages.

15. A  The placental membrane (barrier) may be defined as the fetal tissues which are interposed between the fetal and maternal placental circulations. The structure and thickness of the membrane vary at different stages of pregnancy. The placental membrane becomes extremely thin as pregnancy advances, and increases in permeability. The thickness of the membrane is also affected by the extent of distention of capillaries in the villus.

16. E  Deoxygenated fetal blood passes from the fetus in the umbilical arteries. These arteries divide into a number of radially disposed vessels as the cord attaches to the placenta. The arterial branches pass into the chorionic villi and form an extensive arterio-capillary-venous system.

17. D  Syncytial knots consist of aggregations of nuclei in protuberances of cytoplasm of the syncytiotrophoblast. They form at intervals along a villus; occasionally they break off and enter the maternal circulation. Apparently these nuclear aggregations have a short life in the maternal blood.

18. B  Fibrinoid material develops as a homogeneous layer at various places on the maternal aspect of the villi. As it is at the fetomaternal junction of tissues, fibrinoid is believed to be important in the prevention of rejection of the fetus by the mother. Composed of fibrin and other unidentified substances, fibrinoid decreases the permeability of the placental membrane of the surface area for exchange of material between the fetal and maternal blood streams.

19. C  The amnion adheres to the smooth fetal surface of the placenta, and is continuous with the epithelial membrane covering the umbilical cord. The umbilical vessels radiate over the fetal surface of the placenta deep to the amnion.

20. B  The cytotrophoblast layer (Langhans' layer) begins to retrogress and disappear at about 20 weeks. Some cells of this layer, however, persist until full term.

21. E  Cotyledons are characteristic features of the maternal surface of the placenta. The placental septa divide the maternal surface into 15 to 30 of these areas which give the expelled placenta a cobblestone appearance. During examination of the placenta after delivery, special attention should be given to determining whether the cotyledons are all present and intact. If they are not all recognizable and complete, placental tissue may still be in the uterus and will have to be removed.

22. D  When the umbilical cord and vessels are attached to the margin of the placenta, it is called a battledore placenta because of its resemblance to the bat used in the medieval game of battledore and shuttlecock. This is a common variation of placental form. Battledore placenta (marginal insertion of the cord) has some clinical significance because slight bleeding occasionally occurs. It has also been shown that patients with battledore placenta often have premature labor.

23. B  The cytotrophoblast consists of large, pale cells with relatively large nuclei. Their cytoplasm contains vacuoles and some glycogen. The placenta synthesizes glycogen in early pregnancy, and its declining ability to perform this activity later in pregnancy may be related to the assumption of this function by the fetal liver, and to the retrogression of the cytotrophoblast.

24. A  The main means of attachment of the conceptus to the uterus is by anchoring villi which pass from the chorionic plate to the decidua basalis. Columns of cytotrophoblast cells extend through the syncytiotrophoblast at the tips of these villi and cover the maternal tissue. Soon cytotrophoblast cells from adjacent villi join to form a cytotrophoblastic shell around the conceptus. This shell is also attached to the decidua basalis.

---

NOTES:

# THE CAUSES OF HUMAN CONGENITAL MALFORMATIONS

## O B J E C T I V E S

BE ABLE TO:

---

o   Discuss congenital malformations with special reference to the critical period of development.

o   Define the terms 'teratology' and 'teratogens'.

o   Discuss the causes of congenital malformations under each of the following headings, giving examples of their characteristic malformation patterns:

<u>Genetic Factors</u>: Changes in chromosome number (aneuploidy and polyploidy), structural abnormalities (translocation and deletion), and gene mutation.

<u>Environmental Factors</u>: Irradiation, infections, and drugs.

<u>Genetic and Environmental Factors</u>: Multifactorial inheritance.

---

## F I V E - C H O I C E   C O M P L E T I O N   Q U E S T I O N S

DIRECTIONS: Each of the following statements or questions is followed by five suggested responses or completions. SELECT THE ONE BEST ANSWER in each case and then circle the appropriate letter at the right of each question.

1.   Major congenital malformations are present in about ____ percent of newborn infants.

   A.  0.5                     D.  10
   B.  3.0                     E.  15
   C.  6.0                                      A B C D E

2.   What percentage of deaths in the neonatal period may be attributed to major congenital malformations?

   A.  2                       D.  20
   B.  5                       E.  25
   C.  15                                       A B C D E

SELECT THE ONE BEST ANSWER

3. Most major congenital malformations result from

    A. numerical chromosomal abnormalities
    B. structural chromosomal abnormalities
    C. mutant genes
    D. infectious agents
    E. none of the above                                      A B C D E

4. The infectious agent most likely to cause the following
   triad of congenital malformations: heart defects, cataracts
   and deafness is

    A. Toxoplasma gondii           D. rubella virus
    B. varicella (chickenpox)      E. cytomegalovirus
    C. herpes zoster virus                                    A B C D E

5. Each of the following microorganisms is known to cause major
   congenital malformations except:

    A. Treponema pallidum
    B. cytomegalovirus
    C. varicella
    D. Toxoplasma gondii
    E. rubella virus                                          A B C D E

6. The frequency, severity, and type of abnormalities produced
   by the rubella virus usually depend on the

    A. number of previous infections
    B. mother's age
    C. severity of the infection
    D. time of maternal infection
    E. sex and age of the embryo                              A B C D E

7. Sex chromatin studies indicate that the frequency of sex
   chromatin-positive males in the general population is about
   1:500. Chromosome studies reveal that the most common chromosome complement (karyotype) in these males is

    A. 48,XXXY                     D. 49,XXXYY
    B. 47,XXY                      E. 49,XXXXY
    C. 48,XXYY                                                A B C D E

8. Late maternal age and nondisjunction of chromosomes during
   gametogenesis are often related. In which of the following
   syndromes is late maternal age believed to be a major factor?

    A. Cri du chat syndrome        D. Edwards syndrome
    B. Turner syndrome             E. Down syndrome
    C. Klinefelter syndrome                                   A B C D E

## SELECT THE ONE BEST ANSWER

9. Congenital malformations resulting from chromosomal breakage
   are likely to occur in infants born to mothers who received
   or used:

   A. lysergic acid (LSD)        D. radiation
   B. marijuana                  E. none of the above
   C. heroin                                              A B C D E

10. Certain chemical agents exhibit varying degrees of terato-
    genicity when administered during the embryonic period. Which
    of the following substances is most likely to cause congenital
    malformations in human embryos?

    A. Cortisone                 D. Lysergic acid
    B. Aminopterin               E. Aspirin
    C. Potassium iodide                                   A B C D E

11. Infants with microcephaly are grossly retarded because brain
    development is rudimentary. The cause of this condition is
    often uncertain. Known causes of microcephaly include each
    of the following except:

    A. rubella virus             D. therapeutic radiation
    B. cytomegalovirus           E. thalidomide
    C. Toxoplasma gondii                                  A B C D E

12. Environmental causes of human congenital malformations may be
    prevented to some extent with proper counselling. Each of the
    following would be good advice to give a woman who has just
    missed a menstrual period and may be pregnant, except:

    A. Take only those drugs that have been prescribed by your doctor.
    B. Avoid exposure to large amounts of radiation.
    C. Obtain a vaccination for protection against rubella
       infection.
    D. Stay away from persons with infectious diseases.
    E. Eat a good quality diet and do not smoke.          A B C D E

======================= ANSWERS, NOTES, AND EXPLANATIONS =========================

1. B  It is difficult to obtain an accurate estimate of the incidence of congenital malformations, but it is generally accepted that about 2.7 to 3.0 percent have a medically significant (i.e., major) congenital malformation. If
   one includes minor abnormalities, the incidence is about 5 percent. Not all
   malformations are recognized at birth; indeed if one includes all medically
   significant malformations that are recognized by the end of the first year,
   the incidence increases to over six percent. This emphasizes that less than
   half of all major malformations are detected at birth.

2.  D  About 20 percent of deaths in the neonatal period can be attributed to the presence of congenital malformations (e.g., cardiac malformations and malformations of the central nervous system). More deaths occur in the first month of life than in the remaining months of the first year. Many abnormal embryos can survive before birth, but are unable to adjust to the profound changes associated with the onset of extrauterine life. Failure of the normal changes to occur in the circulatory system results in two of the most common congenital abnormalities of the heart and great vessels (patent foramen ovale and patent ductus arteriosus). In many cases these abnormalities can be corrected by surgical techniques.

3.  E  Most congenital malformations result from unknown causes. Probably most of them are caused by an interaction of genetic and environmental factors (multifactorial inheritance). About 25 percent of malformations are caused by genetic factors (choices A, B, and C), and the remaining malformations are caused by environmental agents such as the rubella virus and drugs.

4.  D  Rubella virus is a potent teratogen if present during early pregnancy. About 20 percent of mothers infected with rubella virus during the first month of pregnancy give birth to malformed infants. This is understandable because the heart, eyes, and internal ears are developing at this time. The risk of malformations from infections during the second and third trimesters is low, but functional defects of the nervous system (e.g., mental retardation) and the internal ears may result from infections as late as the twenty-fifth week.

5.  C  Varicella virus is known to cross the placenta and infect the fetus. No maternal antibodies confer immunity on the fetus as occurs for smallpox. The other microorganisms listed all produce major congenital malformations. Rubella virus produces its effects mainly during the embryonic period, whereas syphilis, cytomegalovirus, and the parasite Toxoplasma gondii all produce their effects during the fetal period.

6.  D  The timing of the rubella infection is the most important factor. Infections early in pregnancy cause the most serious defects. Thus, the extent of damage to the embryo varies with the timing of the maternal infection. Severe infections of the mother early in pregnancy often result in abortion, and milder infections may result in congenital malformations.

7.  B  Newborn males with this chromosomal abnormality appear normal. By puberty they develop the Klinefelter syndrome: small testes and hyalinization of the seminiferous tubules. Usually secondary sexual characteristics are poorly developed, and many of these males are tall and eunuchoid. Subnormal mentality is common especially in persons with more than three sex chromosomes. The chromosomal error (nondisjunction) resulting in the Klinefelter syndrome usually occurs during the first meiotic division of maternal oogenesis, but it can occur during paternal spermatogenesis. In males with four X-chromosomes, nondisjunction occurs during the first and second meiotic divisions.

8.  E  It is well established that the frequency of Down syndrome increases with maternal age. As far as is known, late paternal age has little effect on

nondisjunction. The frequency of this chromosomal error in mothers may be related to the circumstance that the primary oocytes are formed before birth, and remain in the first meiotic prophase until just before ovulation. There is no major maternal-age effect in the other syndromes listed.

9.  D Most structural abnormalities result from chromosome breaks induced by various environmental agents, especially large doses of radiation. Certain viruses have also been shown to cause fragmentation of chromosomes, but there is no conclusive evidence that these chromosomal aberrations produced congenital malformations. Similarly, it is known that LSD and marijuana can cause chromosome damage, but there is not conclusive evidence to indicate that these drugs are teratogenic. Heroin is not known to cause chromosome breakage, but it often causes narcotic addiction in newborn infants.

10. B Aminopterin is a potent teratogen, as are other tumor-inhibiting chemicals (e.g., methotrexate). Potassium iodide may cause congenital goiter and the other substances listed may be weak teratogens, but there is not enough evidence to warrant inclusion of them in a list of known teratogens.

11. E Thalidomide is a highly potent teratogen, producing limb malformations, deafness, and malformations of the cardiovascular and digestive systems, but it does not produce microcephaly, mental retardation or other defects of the central nervous system. All the other environmental agents listed are known to cause microcephaly.

12. C It would be poor advice to recommend vaccination during early pregnancy for any disease. Although there is no conclusive information about the teratogenic potential of live attenuated rubella virus, it is generally contraindicated. Women should be immunized with live attenuated virus only when pregnancy is not planned during the following two months.


# M U L T I - C O M P L E T I O N   Q U E S T I O N S


DIRECTIONS: In each of the following questions or incomplete statements ONE OR MORE of the completions is correct. At the lower right of each question, circle A if 1, 2, and 3 are correct; B if 1 and 3 are correct; C if 2 and 4 are correct; D if only 4 is correct; and E if all are correct.


1.  Sex chromatin tests using buccal smears are useful diagnostic aids for the differential diagnosis of patients with ambiguous sex development, or sterility problems, or retarded mental development. Reliable information these tests provide concerning the sex chromosome complement includes

    1.  the number of X-chromosomes
    2.  anomalies of the Y-chromosome
    3.  monosomy of a sex chromosome
    4.  structural abnormalities                      A B C D E

| A | B | C | D | E |
|---|---|---|---|---|
| 1,2,3 | 1,3 | 2,4 | only 4 | all correct |

2.  Numerical chromosomal abnormalities are common in newborn in-
    fants.  Which of the following chromosome complements usually
    produce recognizable external congenital malformations?

    1.  45,XO                      3.  47, XX
    2.  47,XXX                     4.  47,XXY                    A B C D E

3.  Numerical chromosomal abnormalities may be associated with
    severe mental retardation.  Syndromes that usually exhibit
    this condition include:

    1.  Down syndrome (trisomy 21)
    2.  Turner syndrome (45,XO)
    3.  Edwards syndrome (trisomy 18)
    4.  Klinefelter syndrome (47,XXY)                            A B C D E

4.  It is well established that teratogenic agents produce con-
    genital malformations during the

    1.  fetal period
    2.  first two weeks of development
    3.  organogenetic period
    4.  implantation period                                     A B C D E

5.  Constant characteristics of males with the Klinefelter
    syndrome include:

    1.  gynecomastia
    2.  small testes
    3.  severe mental retardation
    4.  hyalinization of the seminiferous tubules               A B C D E

6.  A laboratory report states that chromatin-positive nuclei
    are present in the oral epithelial cells of a buccal smear;
    the smear could have been taken from a

    1.  47,XYY male
    2.  female with the Down syndrome
    3.  female with the Turner syndrome
    4.  47,XXY male                                             A B C D E

7.  Drugs and chemicals regarded as strong human teratogens
    include:

    1.  methotrexate
    2.  aminopterin
    3.  ethisterone
    4.  thalidomide                                             A B C D E

84

| A | B | C | D | E |
|---|---|---|---|---|
| 1,2,3 | 1,3 | 2,4 | only 4 | all correct |

8. Drugs for which there is strong suggestive evidence of teratogenicity include:

    1. cortisone               3. insulin
    2. aspirin                 4. trimethadione      A B C D E

9. Variables known to affect the recurrent risk of a specific malformation include:

    1. genetic factors        3. season of the year
    2. geographic distribution    4. maternal age       A B C D E

10. Infectious diseases shown to be important in the causation of congenital malformations in human embryos include:

    1. cytomegalic inclusion disease    3. toxoplasmosis
    2. rubeola (measles)             4. influenza         A B C D E

11. Congenital malformations are caused by

    1. chromosomal aberrations    3. infectious agents
    2. multifactorial inheritance    4. drugs and chemicals   A B C D E

12. A newborn infant was observed to have a low birth weight and bilateral congenital cataracts. Subsequently a patent ductus arteriosus was detected and the infant was found to be deaf. Probable causes of these malformations include:

    1. malnutrition and maternal smoking
    2. toxoplasmosis during the second trimester
    3. diagnostic x-rays during the second trimester
    4. German measles during the first trimester      A B C D E

======================== ANSWERS, NOTES, AND EXPLANATIONS ========================

1. B **1 and 3 are correct.** Various sex chromatin patterns are associated with abnormal sex chromosome complexes. Sex chromatin tests give reliable information about cells that have 44 autosomes and variants of XX or XY sex chromosome complex. Tests are available for detecting the Y-chromosome using fluorescence techniques, but they are not routine tests and anomalies of the Y-chromosomes are not detectible using this technique. It is well established that the number of sex chromatin masses is one less than the number of X-chromosomes present, e.g., females with three X-chromosomes (triple-X females) exhibit two masses of sex chromatin in some of their cells. Triple X-females are physically normal and fertile. Their children also appear normal.

2. **B** <u>**1 and 3 are correct**</u>. Newborn triple-X females (47,XXX) and XXY males (47,XXY) usually have no visible congenital malformations. Some of these females are retarded and have a variety of nonspecific and minor congenital anomalies which do not appear to be related to the chromosomal abnormality. The XXY males appear normal at birth, but by puberty their testes undergo atrophy (absence of germ cells and testicular fibrosis). These males often become tall and eunuchoid. Females with the 45,XO chromosome complement develop Turner syndrome or gonadal dysgenesis; newborns often show webbing of the neck and marked lymphedema of the feet. Persons with 47,XX (or 47,XY), i.e., an extra autosome, have severe abnormalities; the most common is Down syndrome.

3. **B** <u>**1 and 3 are correct**</u>. Infants with Turner syndrome usually have normal intelligence. Newborn infants with the usual 47,XXY chromosomal abnormality appear normal at birth and their mental defect, if any, is usually not detectible during infancy. Subnormal mentality may be detected later in these males, but it is not severe. Usually males with Klinefelter syndrome associated with four or more sex chromosomes (e.g., 49,XXXXY) are severely retarded. Infants with typical Down syndrome (trisomy 21) and Edwards syndrome (trisomy 18) are always mentally retarded. Infants with trisomy 18 have more severe congenital malformations than those with trisomy 21, and the mental defect is much greater. Most infants with trisomy 18 die by the age of six months.

4. **B** <u>**1 and 3 are correct**</u>. Development is most easily disturbed during the organogenetic period (i.e., when the organs are forming). Development of the external genitalia can be disturbed during the eighth and ninth weeks, and microcephaly and microphthalmia can result from disturbance by microorganisms in the second trimester. Teratogens acting during the first two weeks, which includes the implantation period, are not known to cause malformations. Environmental agents acting during this period may, however, kill the embryo, prevent implantation, or cause chromosomal abnormalities.

5. **C** <u>**2 and 4 are correct**</u>. Small testes and hyalinization of the seminiferous tubules are constant characteristics of chromatin-positive males with Klinefelter syndrome. Usually secondary sexual characteristics are poorly developed and the persons are tall and eunuchoid. Some 47,XXY males develop gynecomastia (enlarged breasts), and subnormal mentality is common. Aspermatogenesis is present in most males with the Klinefelter syndrome. The error in meiosis (nondisjunction) is usually maternal and may occur during the first or second meiotic division.

6. **C** <u>**2 and 4 are correct**</u>. A female with Down syndrome usually has no abnormality of the sex chromosome complex, and therefore has sex chromatin-positive nuclei. Males with Klinefelter syndrome usually have an XXY sex chromosome complex and the extra X chromosome forms sex chromatin in the cells. The sex chromatin pattern is similar to normal males (i.e., chromatin negative) in females with the Turner syndrome and in males with two Y chromosomes. Because only one X is present in their cells, no sex chromatin is visible.

7. **E** <u>**All are correct**</u>. All these substances are considered to be teratogenic in

human embryos. Because of the well established teratogenicity of thalidomide, this drug was withdrawn from the market. Aminopterin and methotrexate are tumor-inhibiting chemicals that are known to be highly teratogenic. Ethisterone is a synthetic progestin that is believed to produce varying degrees of masculinization of female fetuses. None of these chemicals should be administered during pregnancy, especially during the organogenetic period.

8.  D  Only 4 is correct. There is strong suggestive evidence that two anti-epileptic drugs, trimethadione (Tridione) and paramethadione (Paradione), may cause facial abnormalities, cardiac defects, cleft palate, and growth retardation. There is little evidence to suggest that cortisone, aspirin, or insulin produce congenital malformations even when given during the organogenetic period. If they are necessary they should be administered with caution during early pregnancy. When maternal medication is strongly indicated (e.g., for diabetes mellitus or epilepsy), it is necessary to consider the possible harmful effects of the drug to the embryo and weigh these against the benefits of the treatment to the mother.

9.  E  All are correct. Genetic factors are involved in many congenital malformations. Often the same malformations (e.g., cardiac, sexual, and neural tube defects) occur in more than one member of the family. Meroanencephly (anencephaly) shows a striking variation in geographic distribution, e.g., it is more than 50 times as common in Belfast as in Lyons. It is well established that persons with the Down syndrome are born more often to older mothers. The maternal age factor is less important in the etiology of the Klinefelter syndrome. It should be emphasized that the father's age appears not to be a factor in most cases of congenital malformation. The season of the year also seems to be a factor in some malformations, e.g., the risk of meroanencephaly is many times higher for girls in Belfast in winter, than for boys in Lyons in summer.

10. B  1 and 3 are correct. Unlike rubella (German measles), rubeola or common measles does not cause congenital malformations in human embryos. Maternal antibodies are known to cross the placenta and confer immunity on the embryo to rubeola, diphtheria, and smallpox. Influenza and mumps have often been suspected of being teratogens, but there is insufficient evidence to implicate these infections as causes of human malformations. Cytomegalic inclusion disease caused by the Toxoplasma gondii intracellular parasite has been proved beyond all doubt to be important in the causation of congenital malformations, especially microcephaly, hydrocephalus, and microphthalmia.

11. E  All are correct. About 65 percent of congenital malformations are caused by unknown factors, probably a combination of genetic and environmental factors. About 25 percent of malformations can be attributed to genetic factors, and no more than 10 percent are believed to result from environmental factors such as infectious agents, drugs, and chemicals.

12. D  Only 4 is correct. The case described is a typical brief history of a baby with the congenital rubella syndrome. These abnormalities would not be caused by the Toxoplasma microorganism or by diagnostic x-ray examinations of the mother. Malnutrition and heavy smoking by the mother could cause low birth weight. However, in severe rubella infection, growth retardation is a common finding at birth.

# FIVE-CHOICE ASSOCIATION QUESTIONS

DIRECTIONS: Each group of questions below consists of a numbered list of descriptive words or phrases accompanied by a diagram with certain parts indicated by letters, or by a list of lettered headings. For each numbered word or phrase, SELECT THE LETTERED PART OR HEADING that matches it correctly. Then insert the letter in the space to the right of the appropriate number. Sometimes more than one numbered word or phrase may be correctly matched to the same lettered part or heading.

A. 47,XXX
B. 45,XO
C. Trisomy 18

D. Trisomy 21
E. 47,XXY

1. B   Webbed neck and short stature
2. C   Mental retardation, low set ears, and early postnatal death
3. A   Normal female appearance and usually fertile
4. E   Small testes and hyalinization of the seminiferous tubules
5. D   The most common numerical autosomal abnormality
6. B   Female with sex chromatin-negative nuclei
7. D   Strong associatiion with late maternal age
8. D   Mental retardation, simian crease, and heart defect
9. E   Sterile male with sex chromatin-positive nuclei

A. Cytomegalovirus
B. Androgenic agents
C. Thalidomide

D. Toxoplasma gondii
E. Aminopterin

10. E   An antitumor agent and potent teratogen
11. D   An intracellular parasite that is found in cats
12. C   A potent teratogen that affects limb development
13. B   May cause masculinization of female fetuses
14. E   Known to cause meroanencephaly (anencephaly)
15. D   Mother may contract it by eating poorly cooked meat

======================= ANSWERS, NOTES, AND EXPLANATIONS =========================

1. B  Webbed neck and short stature are associated with females with the Turner syndrome (ovarian dysgenesis). These persons have 44 autosomes and only one X-chromosome. In the newborn period, these infants usually exhibit marked edema of the feet and webbing of the neck. The ovaries usually consist of only connective tissue streaks. Many of these girls are not recognized until

they reach puberty (12-15 years), at which time they seek medical advice about primary amenorrhea (failure of menstruation to begin) and the lack of secondary sex development.

2.  C  Infants with trisomy 18 (also called E syndrome and Edwards syndrome) have multiple major malformations. Like those with the less common trisomy 13 syndrome, these infants have a severe mental defect and they die during early infancy. Trisomy 18 is much more severe than Down syndrome, and an excess of females are affected (about 78 percent).

3.  A  Females with the triple X chromosome abnormality usually appear normal and are fertile. These women have two sex chromatin masses in their cells because of the presence of the extra X-chromosome. Some triple X females have borne children, all of whom are normal and have normal karyotypes. Females with four or more X-chromosomes are also usually physically normal, but they are often severely retarded.

4.  E  XXY males appear normal at birth. Small testes and hyalinization of the seminiferous tubules are the constant characteristics of postpubertal XXY males with the Klinefelter syndrome. The secondary sexual characteristics are usually poorly developed and many of these males are tall and eunuchoid. Subnormal mentality is very common.

5.  D  Trisomy 21 is the most common type of numerical autosomal abnormality, occurring about once in 600 newborn infants. The cause of the chromosomal abnormality (trisomy of chromosome 21) is nondisjunction during oogenesis, usually in older mothers. About four percent of persons with the Down syndrome have the extra 21 chromosome attached to another chromosome (usually number 14).

6.  B  Females with the Turner syndrome (45,XO) were among the first cases studied when accurate chromosome analyses became possible in 1958. Sex chromatin studies had shown a few years earlier that these females had chromatin-negative nuclei. Some females with stigmata of the Turner syndrome are chromatin positive because they are mosaics (i.e., they have a 45,X cell line and a normal 46,XX cell line).

7.  D  It is well known that infants with the Down syndrome are more often born to older mothers. The mean maternal age is about 35 years compared with 28 in a control population. The older name for this condition was mongolism, coined because of the somewhat oriental slant of the eyes. It is an inappropriate name and should not be used.

8.  D  Infants with the Down syndrome are mentally retarded (I.Q. is usually in the 25 to 50 range) and have a heart defect. The single transverse crease (simian crease) in place of the usual creases is found in about 50 percent of persons with the syndrome. It is also found in persons with other chromosomal abnormalities, and in about one percent of apparently normal persons. It is important to realize therefore that the presence of a simian crease does not necessarily indicate a chromosomal abnormality and the Down syndrome, but it is a useful criterion when associated with other typical characteristics (hypotonia, epicanthal folds, furrowed and protruding tongue).

9. E Males with sex chromatin-positive nuclei have the Klinefelter syndrome or a related condition. Newborn males appear normal but the testes remain abnormally small as puberty approaches owing to hyalinization of the seminiferous tubules. Consequently they are sterile. Secondary sexual characteristics develop poorly and gynecomastia (enlargement of the breasts) may occur. Usually these men are tall and eunuchoid and commonly have a subnormal mentality.

10. E Aminopterin, an antitumor agent, is also a potent human teratogen. Methotrexate, a derivative of aminopterin, is also teratogenic. These agents produce a wide range of severe skeletal defects and malformations of the central nervous system. Aminopterin may produce meroanencephaly (anencephaly), intrauterine growth retardation, and many other abnormalities.

11. D Toxoplasma gondii is a protozoan, intracellular parasite. It infects many birds and mammals, in addition to man. Toxoplasmosis, the disease caused by this microorganism, can be contracted from eating raw meat or through contact with infected animals. This parasite affects the fetus during the second and third trimesters, producing microcephaly, microphthalmia, hydrocephaly, and chorioretinitis.

12. C Thalidomide has been shown to produce severe malformations in the embryo if taken by the mother during the first trimester. As little as 200 mg of this sedative and antinauseant may cause limb defects, cardiac malformations, and ear anomalies.

13. B Androgenic agents and certain progestins administered to prevent abortion may cause masculinization of female fetuses. The substances known to cause these malformations are ethisterone and norethisterone. All substances with known androgenic properties may cause masculinization if administered during the first trimester of pregnancy.

14. E Aminopterin, an antitumor agent, is known to cause anencephaly or meroanencephaly (absence or partial absence of the brain) if administered during the early period of brain development (third to fourth weeks after fertilization).

15. D A mother may become infected with the parasite, Toxoplasma gondii, by eating raw or poorly-cooked meat containing the microorganism. She may contract the disease, toxoplasmosis, from infected birds, animals or persons. If the parasite crosses the placental membrane, it causes maldevelopment during the fetal period. It causes microcephaly, microphthalmia, hydrocephaly, and chorioretinitis. There is no proof that the parasite affects development during organogenesis, i.e., during the embryonic period.

NOTES:

# BODY CAVITIES, PRIMITIVE MESENTERIES AND THE DIAPHRAGM

## O B J E C T I V E S

BE ABLE TO:

o   Describe, with the aid of diagrams, the development of the intra-embryonic coelom and the changes resulting in it from longitudinal and transverse folding of the embryo during the fourth week.

o   Give an account of the subdivision or partitioning of the body cavities into: (1) the pericardial cavity, (2) the pleural cavities, and (3) the peritoneal cavity.

o   Explain, with the aid of diagrams, the formation of the dorsal and ventral mesenteries.

o   Construct and label diagrams showing the development of the diaphragm. Discuss its four components, positional changes, and innervation.

o   Explain the embryological basis of congenital diaphragmatic hernia. Discuss the possible effects of this defect on the initiation of respiration at birth.

## F I V E - C H O I C E   C O M P L E T I O N   Q U E S T I O N S

DIRECTIONS: Each of the following statements or questions is followed by five suggested responses or completions. SELECT THE ONE BEST ANSWER in each case and then circle the appropriate letter at the right of each question.

1. Each of the following structures is involved in the development of the diaphragm except the

   A. lateral body wall
   B. pleuroperitoneal membranes
   C. septum transversum
   D. pleuropericardial membranes
   E. esophageal mesentery

   A B C D E

2. The intraembryonic coelom (embryonic body cavity) is first recognizable during the ____ week after fertilization.

   A. second
   B. third
   C. fourth
   D. fifth
   E. sixth

   A B C D E

SELECT THE ONE BEST ANSWER

3.  The first component of the developing diaphragm is recognizable at the end of the ____ week of development.

    A.  second            D.  fifth
    B.  third             E.  sixth
    C.  fourth                                          A B C D E

4.  After folding of the embryo, the dorsal mesentery extends from the

    A.  cranial part of the foregut to the caudal region of the hindgut
    B.  caudal part of the foregut to the cranial part of the hindgut
    C.  caudal part of the esophagus to the cloacal region
    D.  cranial part of the esophagus to the cloacal region
    E.  stomodeum to the proctodeum                      A B C D E

5.  Failure of closure of the cranial end of the pericardioperitoneal canal results in communication between the pleural cavity on the affected side and the

    A.  peritoneal cavity       D.  other pleural cavity
    B.  pericardial cavity      E.  pelvic cavity
    E.  abdominopelvic cavity                            A B C D E

6.  Failure of closure of the caudal end of the pericardioperitoneal canal results in communication between the pleural cavity on the affected side and the

    A.  peritoneal cavity       D.  other pleural cavity
    B.  pericardial cavity      E.  pelvic cavity
    E.  abdominopelvic cavity                            A B C D E

7.  In the four-week embryo, the developing diaphragm (represented by the septum transversum) is located at the level of the

    A.  superior cervical somites
    B.  inferior thoracic somites
    C.  superior thoracic somites                        A B C D E
    D.  superior lumbar somites
    E.  inferior lumbar somites

8.  Most muscle-forming cells (myoblasts) giving rise to the musculature of the diaphragm are derived from mesenchymal cells that originate in the

    A.  septum transversum      D.  lumbar somites
    B.  cervical somites        E.  lateral mesoderm
    C.  thoracic somites                                 A B C D E

92

SELECT THE ONE BEST ANSWER

9. The septum transversum gives rise to ____ of the diaphragm.

    A. small intermediate portions
    B. the right and left crura
    C. the central tendon

    D. posterolateral portions
    E. peripheral portions

    A B C D E

10. In the five-week embryo, the ventral mesentery of the primitive gut disappears, except where it is attached to the:

    A. primitive pharynx
    B. embryonic part of the yolk stalk
    C. caudal region of the hindgut
    D. caudal region of the foregut
    E. cranial region of the midgut

    A B C D E

======================= ANSWERS, NOTES, AND EXPLANATIONS =========================

1. D  The other four structures listed are the main components of the developing diaphragm. The pleuropericardial membranes are not involved in the formation of the diaphragm. They form partitions at the cranial ends of the pericardioperitoneal canals and separate the pericardial cavity from the pleural cavities.

2. B  Intercellular spaces, lined by mesothelium, appear in the lateral mesoderm, and in the cardiogenic mesoderm, 18-19 days after fertilization. These spaces coalesce to form the intraembryonic coelom, a horseshoe-shaped cavity within the lateral mesoderm and cardiogenic mesoderm of the trilaminar embryonic disc.

3. B  The septum transversum is the first recognizable component of the developing diaphragm. It appears at the end of the third week as a mass of mesoderm, cranial to the pericardial coelom. After the head fold occurs during the fourth week, the septum transversum forms a thick mass of mesenchyme between the thoracic and abdominopelvic cavities. Later it becomes extensively invaded by the developing liver and eventually becomes a thin layer (the primordium of the central tendon) between the pericardial cavity and the liver.

4. C  The dorsal mesentery extends from the caudal part (inferior end) of the esophagus to the cloacal region of the hindgut. In the region of the esophagus, the mesentery is called the mesoesophagus; in the stomach region it is called the dorsal mesogastrium or greater omentum; and in the region of the colon, it is called mesocolon. The dorsal mesentery of the jejunum and ileum is called the mesentery proper. The dorsal mesentery of the duodenum (dorsal mesoduodenum) disappears completely, except in the region of the

93

pylorus of the stomach.

5.  B  Defective formation and/or fusion of the pleuropericardial membrane, usually on the left side, is uncommon. When this occurs there is a defect in the fibrous pericardium, the adult derivative of the pleuropericardial membranes. Part of the left atrium may herniate into the left pleural cavity if there is a defect in the pericardium.

6.  A  Defective formation and/or fusion of the pleuroperitoneal membrane, usually on the left side, is relatively common (occurs about once in 2000 births). This results in a posterolateral defect in the diaphragm through which abdominal viscera may herniate into the thorax. Congenital diaphragmatic hernia usually constitutes a medical-surgical emergency in the newborn period because of respiratory disorders (pressure on the lungs causing poor lung expansion and difficult breathing).

7.  A  As the head fold forms, the septum transversum and the pericardial cavity swing into a ventral position. When it lies opposite to the upper cervical segments of the spinal cord, nerves from the third, fourth, and fifth segments grow into the septum transversum forming the phrenic nerves. These nerves are the sole motor nerve supply to the diaphragm and they are also sensory to the central part of the diaphragm derived from the septum transversum. In the later weeks of development, the diaphragm descends so that the dorsal part reaches the level of the first lumbar vertebra by the end of the embryonic period.

8.  B  Most of the musculature of the diaphragm is thought to be derived from mesenchymal cells that originate in the myotome regions of the cervical somites. When these cells migrate into the septum transversum with the developing phrenic nerves, they differentiate into myoblasts (developing muscle fibers). When the developing diaphragm migrates caudally during subsequent development, the phrenic nerves supplying these muscles follow the diaphragm caudally. Some myoblasts probably differentiate from mesenchymal cells in the septum transversum. Other myoblasts likely arise from mesenchymal cells that migrate from the thoracic somites and enter the diaphragm with the lateral body wall tissues that split off when the pleural cavities enlarge into the chest wall.

9.  C  The septum transversum gives rise to the central tendon of the diaphragm. Small intermediate portions of it are derived from the pleuroperitoneal membranes, and the crura develop from the growth of muscle fibers into the dorsal mesentery of the esophagus. The peripheral portions of the diaphragm are derived from lateral body wall tissue that is split off as the lungs and pleural cavities enlarge and burrow into the lateral body walls.

10. D  The ventral mesentery disappears except where it is attached to the caudal (inferior) part of the foregut. This region gives rise to the terminal portion of the esophagus, the stomach, and the superior part of the duodenum. Caudal to the bile duct, the intestines have no ventral mesentery. When most of the ventral mesentery disappears, the right and left peritoneal cavities become a continuous large peritoneal sac in which the viscera are suspended by the dorsal mesentery.

# MULTI-COMPLETION QUESTIONS

DIRECTIONS: In each of the following questions or incomplete statements ONE OR MORE of the completions is correct. At the lower right of each question, circle A if 1, 2, and 3 are correct; B if 1 and 3 are correct; C if 2 and 4 are correct; D if only 4 is correct; and E if all are correct.

1. A congenital diaphragmatic hernia through a posterolateral defect of the diaphragm usually results from a failure of the left pleuroperitoneal membrane to fuse with the

   1. right pleuroperitoneal membrane
   2. dorsal mesentery of the esophagus
   3. fibrous pericardium
   4. septum transversum                          A B C D E

2. Correct statements about a congenital diaphragmatic hernia through a posterolateral defect of the diaphragm include:

   1. It is the most common type of congenital diaphragmatic hernia.
   2. The stomach, intestines, and part of the liver may herniate into the thoracic cavity.
   3. It occurs more often on the left side than the right.
   4. The lungs are often compressed and hypoplastic.    A B C D E

3. The diaphragm is a musculomembranous partition between the thoracic and abdominal cavities. Structures contributing to its development are the

   1. body wall
   2. dorsal mesoesophagus
   3. septum transversum
   4. pleuropericardial membranes                 A B C D E

4. In which position(s) might you observe the dorsal part of the diaphragm during the embryonic period of its development?

   1. Fifth cervical
   2. Fifth thoracic
   3. Eighth thoracic
   4. First lumbar                                 A B C D E

5. For a teratogen to produce a posterolateral defect of the diaphragm, it would likely act:

   1. on the developing musculature
   2. on a pleuroperitoneal membrane
   3. before the end of the sixth week
   4. on the septum transversum                    A B C D E

| A | B | C | D | E |
|---|---|---|---|---|
| 1,2,3 | 1,3 | 2,4 | only 4 | all correct |

6. By the end of the sixth week, the embryonic diaphragm forms a complete partition between the thoracic and abdominal cavities. At this stage, it is composed of contributions from the

    1. pleuroperitoneal membranes
    2. esophageal mesentery
    3. septum transversum
    4. dorsal body wall
                                                       A B C D E

7. Correct statements concerning innervation of the developing diaphragm include:

    1. The phrenic nerves pass to the diaphragm via the pleuro-pericardial membranes.
    2. The sole motor nerve supply of the diaphragm is from the third, fourth, and fifth cervical segments of the spinal cord.
    3. Marginal branches are supplied to the diaphragm by intercostal nerves.
    4. The phrenic nerves form during the eighth week as the diaphragm descends.
                                                         A B C D E

8. Congenital pericardial defects are uncommon and result in communication between the pericardial and pleural cavities. The usual embryological basis for these defects is a failure of the left pleuropericardial membrane to fuse with the

    1. septum transversum
    2. right pleuroperitoneal membrane
    3. dorsal mesentery of the esophagus
    4. mesoderm ventral to the esophagus
                                                   A B C D E

9. The pleuropericardial membranes give rise to the fibrous pericardium of the adult heart. In the embryo, each of these membranes contains a

    1. developing lung
    2. cardinal vein
    3. pleural canal
    4. phrenic nerve
                                                   A B C D E

10. After folding of the embryo and formation of the primitive mesenteries, structures suspended in the peritoneal cavity by the dorsal mesentery include:

    1. caudal part of foregut        3. midgut loop
    2. hindgut                    4. allantois          A B C D E

======================== ANSWERS, NOTES, AND EXPLANATIONS ==========================

1. C  2 and 4 are correct.  A left posterolateral defect in the diaphragm results when the left pleuroperitoneal membrane fails to fuse with the dorsal mesentery of the esophagus and the dorsal part of the septum transversum.  A posterolateral diaphragmatic defect could also result from failure of a pleuroperitoneal membrane to form.  There are two other kinds of congenital diaphragmatic defect (hiatal and retrosternal), but they are uncommon.

2. E  All are correct.  This type of congenital diaphragmatic hernia occurs about once in every 2000 births; the other two types of congenital diaphragmatic hernia are uncommon.  The intestines may enter the thorax through the defect in the diaphragm as they re-enter the abdomen from the umbilical cord during the tenth week. Occasionally the stomach and large bowel also pass into the thorax.  The defect occurs five times more often on the left side than on the right, possibly because the large liver on the right side aids the fusion of the pleuroperitoneal membrane with the other diaphragmatic components.  The presence of the viscera in the thorax often compresses the lungs resulting in difficulty in the initiation and maintenance of breathing.  Occasionally the viscera move freely through the defect, so that they are sometimes in the thoracic cavity and other times in the abdominal cavity, depending on the fetus's position.  In such cases, there may be no symptoms at all at birth, and the defect may be detected first on a chest film taken for other purposes during childhood.

3. A  1, 2, and 3 are correct.  The other structures involved in the development of the diaphragm are the pleuroperitoneal membranes.  The pleuropericardial membranes do not give rise to any part of the diaphragm, but the phrenic nerves pass through them to reach the diaphragm.  When the pleuroperitoneal membranes fuse with the septum transversum and the mesoesophagus, a complete partition is formed between the thoracic and abdominal cavities.  The ingrowth of tissue from the lateral body wall occurs about a month later, completing development of the diaphragm.  The pleuropericardial membranes fuse and separate the pericardial cavity from the pleural cavities and become the fibrous pericardium.

4. E  All are correct.  The diaphragm is first represented by the septum transversum during the early part of the fourth week.  During folding of the head region of the embryo, the developing diaphragm (septum transversum) lies opposite the superior cervical somites.  During the fifth week, nerves from the third to fifth spinal cord segments grow into the developing diaphragm.  By the sixth week the developing diaphragm is at the level of the thoracic segments, and by the end of the embryonic period, the dorsal part of the diaphragm usually lies at the level of the first lumbar vertebra.

5. A  1, 2, and 3 are correct.  A teratogen would have to exert its action before formation of the primitive diaphragm at the end of the sixth week by interfering with the development or fusion or both of the pleuroperitoneal membrane with other diaphragmatic components.  It would probably also affect the production and ingrowth of mesenchyme into the pleuroperitoneal membrane,

and the subsequent development of muscle. If a teratogen acted on the septum transversum, it would probably result in a retrosternal hernia or an eventration of the diaphragm.

6.   A <u>1, 2, and 3 are correct</u>. The pleuroperitoneal membranes fuse with the dorsal mesentery of the esophagus and the dorsal portion of the septum transversum. This completes the partition between the thoracic and abdominal cavities and forms the primitive diaphragm. The contributions to the peripheral portions of the diaphragm from the body wall are added later (ninth to twelfth weeks).

7.   A <u>1, 2, and 3 are correct</u>. The phrenic nerves from the cervical plexus are the sole motor supply of the diaphragm. They also carry sensory fibers from the central portion of the diaphragm. The sensory fibers from the periphery of the diaphragm are in the intercostal nerves which enter peripheral regions of the diaphragm as the lateral body wall contributes to the diaphragm. The phrenic nerves form during the fourth and fifth weeks by the union of branches of the ventral primary rami of the third, fourth, and fifth cervical nerves.

8.   D <u>Only 4 is correct</u>. Defective formation and/or fusion of the left pleuropericardial membrane with the mesoderm ventral to the esophagus (the primitive mediastinum) results in a persistent connection between the pericardial and pleural cavities on the left side. The larger size of the right common cardial vein, producing a larger membrane, is thought to effect earlier closure of this connection between the pericardial and pleural cavities on the right side. Consequently, congenital pericardial defects are almost always on the left side.

9.   C <u>2 and 4 are correct</u>. The pleuropericardial membranes initially appear as ridges or bulges of mesenchyme, each containing a common cardinal vein on its way to the heart. These veins drain the primitive venous system into the heart. The phrenic nerves, from the third to fifth cervical segments, pass through the pleuropericardial membranes on their way to the septum transversum (the first part of the diaphragm to form). Later these membranes become the fibrous pericardium of the heart (external layer of the fibrous sac sheathing the heart). The pleural canals (future pleural cavities) and the developing lungs lie dorsal to the pleuropericardial membranes.

10.  A <u>1, 2, and 3 are correct</u>. The dorsal mesentery extends the full length of the intraabdominal part of the primitive gut. The dorsal mesentery serves as a pathway for the blood vessels, nerves, and lymphatics supplying the gastrointestinal tract. The dorsal mesentery of the stomach grows extensively and soon hangs over the transverse colon and small intestines like an apron, forming the greater omentum. The allantois has no mesentery.

# FIVE-CHOICE ASSOCIATION QUESTIONS

DIRECTIONS: Each group of questions below consists of a numbered list of descriptive words or phrases accompanied by a diagram with certain parts indicated by letters, or by a list of lettered headings. For each numbered word or phrase, SELECT THE LETTERED PART OR HEADING that matches it correctly. Then insert the letter in the space to the right of the appropriate number. Sometimes more than one numbered word or phrase may be correctly matched to the same lettered part or heading.

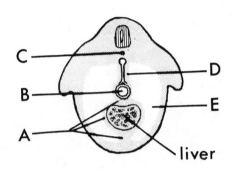

1. __D__  Disappears caudally
2. __E__  Derived from the coelom
3. __A__  Ventral mesentery of the stomach
4. __B__  Caudal part of the foregut
5. __D__  Dorsal mesogastrium

A. Costodiaphragmatic recess
B. Cervical myotomes
C. Congenital hiatal hernia

D. Pleuroperitoneal membrane
E. Pericardioperitoneal canal

6. __C__  Large esophageal opening
7. __A__  Extension of the pleural cavity
8. __D__  Posterolateral diaphragmatic defect
9. __B__  Diaphragmatic muscles
10. __E__  Connects the pericardial and peritoneal cavities
11. __D__  Herniation of the abdominal viscera

99

## ASSOCIATION QUESTIONS

A. Esophageal mesentery
B. Pleuropericardial membrane
C. Phrenic nerves

D. Crura of the diaphragm
E. Embryonic mediastinum

12. _C_ Derived from the third to fifth cervical cord segments
13. _B_ Common cardial vein
14. _D_ Muscular origins of the diaphragm
15. _E_ Mesenchyme separating the lungs
16. _A_ Forms the median portion of the diaphragm

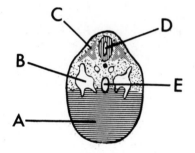

17. _B_ future pleural cavity
18. _E_ gives rise to the esophagus
19. _C_ produces mesenchyme
20. _A_ gives rise to the central tendon
21. _A_ located caudal to the heart

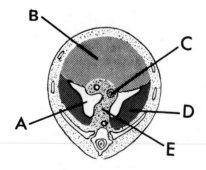

22. _D_ pleuroperitoneal membrane
23. _C_ derived from the foregut
24. _B_ esophageal mesentery
25. _A_ future pleural cavity
26. _E_ gives rise to the central tendon

======================= ANSWERS, NOTES, AND EXPLANATIONS =========================

1.  A  The ventral mesentery disappears caudal to the superior or first part of
    the duodenum.  Note that the liver is developing between the layers of the
    ventral mesentery.  The ventral mesentery forms during transverse folding of
    the embryo and gives rise to: (1) the lesser omentum, (2) the falciform
    ligament, and (3) the visceral peritoneum of the liver.

2.  E  The peritoneal cavity is derived from the caudal extension of the horse-
    shoe-shaped intraembryonic coelom that develops early in the fourth week of
    development.  In the illustration, the foregut (developing stomach) is
    suspended in the peritoneal cavity by the dorsal mesentery (dorsal
    mesogastrium) and the ventral mesentery (hepatogastric ligament).

3.  A  The ventral mesentery (mesogastrium) of the stomach develops from the
    septum transversum and extends from this septum to the ventral aspect of the
    caudal part of the foregut.  This part of the foregut gives rise to the
    stomach and the superior part of the duodenum.  After the liver develops, the
    ventral mesentery attaches the stomach to the liver (hepatogastric ligament)
    and the first part of the duodenum to the liver (hepatoduodenal ligament).

4.  B  The endoderm of the caudal part of the foregut gives rise to the
    epithelium and glands of the inferior end of the esophagus, the stomach, and
    the superior part of the duodenum.  The muscular and fibrous elements of
    these structures are derived from the surrounding splanchnic mesoderm.  The
    superior part of the foregut gives rise to the pharynx and its derivatives,
    the lower respiratory tract, and the superior part of the esophagus.

5.  D  The dorsal mesentery (mesogastrium) of the stomach suspends the stomach in
    the peritoneal cavity.  Subsequently the spleen develops between the two
    layers of the dorsal mesogastrium.  Later, as the result of positional
    changes and growth, the dorsal mesogastrium hangs over the transverse colon
    and the small intestines from which it hangs like an apron; this portion of
    the dorsal mesentery is called the greater omentum.

6.  C  If the embryonic esophageal hiatus or opening in the diaphragm is
    excessively large, abdominal viscera may herniate through it into the thorax,
    producing a congenital hiatal hernia.  Another uncommon type of congenital
    diaphragmatic hernia, the esophageal hernia, is believed to be caused by a
    short esophagus.  Because of this malformation, the superior part of the
    stomach remains in the thorax and the stomach is constricted where it passes
    through the esophageal opening.

7.  A  As the pleural cavities enlarge they extend into the body walls, forming
    costodiaphragmatic recesses.  This 'excavation' process also splits off body
    wall tissue which contributes to peripheral portions of the diaphragm, and
    establishes the characteristic dome-shaped configuration of the diaphragm.

8.  D  If the pleuroperitoneal membrane fails to develop, or to fuse with other
    parts of the diaphragm, a posterolateral defect develops, usually on the left

101

side. Associated with this defect is herniation of abdominal viscera into the thorax and compression of the lungs. This type of congenital diaphragmatic hernia often results in a medical-surgical emergency because of difficulty in breathing.

9. B  The diaphragmatic muscles are mainly derived from myoblasts that migrate from the myotome regions of the cervical somites. Other myoblasts are derived from the myotome regions of the thoracic somites and some myoblasts originate in the body wall tissues.

10. E  The pericardioperitoneal canals give rise to the adult pleural cavities. Membranes develop at the cranial and caudal ends of these canals that separate the pleural cavities from the pericardial cavity and the peritoneal cavity respectively. The developing lungs invaginate the medial walls of the pericardioperitoneal cavities. Eventually the inner (visceral) and outer (parietal) walls of these canals come close together as the layers of pleura.

11. D  Herniation of abdominal viscera into the thorax occurs through a postero-lateral defect in the diaphragm where there is failure of development or fusion of the pleuroperitoneal membrane with other parts of the diaphragm, usually on the left side. Because of the presence of abdominal viscera in the thorax, the lungs are often compressed and may be hypoplastic (incompletely developed).

12. C  The phrenic nerves are derived from the third, fourth, and fifth cervical segments of the spinal cord. These nerves accompany the myoblasts that grow into the developing diaphragm from the myotome regions of the cervical somites. The diaphragm descends as elongation of the neck, descent of the heart, and expansion of the pericardial and pleural cavities occur. Descent of the diaphragm, after it receives its main nerve supply, explains the rather unusual course of the phrenic nerves.

13. B  The common cardinal veins, which are the main venous channels entering the heart, lie in the pleuropericardial membranes. At first these membranes appear as small ridges projecting into the pericardioperitoneal canals. Eventually they fuse with the mesoderm ventral to the esophagus (primitive mediastinum), closing the connections between the pericardial cavity and the pleural cavities.

14. D  The crura of the diaphragm (muscular origins of the diaphragm from the superior lumbar vertebrae) develop as muscle fibers within the esophageal mesentery.

15. E  The mediastinum (median septum) in the embryo consists of a mass of mesenchymal tissue separating the lungs and extending from the sternum to the vertebral column. It forms the median dividing wall of the thoracic cavity and contains all the thoracic viscera and structures except the lungs.

16. A  The dorsal mesentery of the esophagus (mesoesophagus) forms the median portion of the diaphragm. The pleuroperitoneal membranes fuse with the esophageal mesentery and the septum transversum during the sixth week, forming a partition between the thoracic and abdominal cavities. Completion

of the diaphragm occurs during the ninth to twelfth weeks as body wall tissue is added to it peripherally.

17. B  The pericardioperitoneal canals are the future pleural cavities.  As the lungs develop they invaginate (push into) the medial walls of these canals, like fists pushed into the sides of almost empty balloons.  These invaginations are so complete that the space between the two walls of the canals (future layers of pleura) is reduced to a narrow gap.

18. E  The foregut gives rise to the epithelium and glands of the esophagus and stomach.  Other regions of the foregut give rise to the pharynx and its derivatives, the lower respiratory tract, the duodenum as far as the bile duct, the liver, pancreas, and biliary apparatus.

19. C  The somites, derived by division of the paraxial mesoderm, give rise to the mesenchyme that differentiates into most of the axial skeleton and its associated musculature.  Mesenchyme is an embryonic connective tissue that gives rise to a wide variety of adult tissues, e.g., fibroblasts, fibrocytes, osteoblasts, osteocytes, chondroblasts, chondrocytes, myoblasts, muscle fibers, etc.

20. A  The septum transversum, a thick mass of mesenchyme, gives rise to the central tendon of the diaphragm.  It is the first component of the diaphragm to be recognizable (end of 3rd week).  It forms the caudal limit of the pericardial cavity after folding of the embryo and separates it from the future peritoneal cavity.  During the fourth week, groups of myoblasts (muscle-forming cells) from the cervical somites (3 to 5) migrate into the cranial part of the septum transversum, carrying their phrenic nerve fibers with them.

21. A  The septum transversum is located caudal to the heart.  Early in the fourth week, it lies cranial to the pericardial coelom and the developing heart.  As the brain develops, the head folds ventrally carrying the septum transversum, developing heart, pericardial coelom, the oropharyngeal membrane ventral to the foregut.

22. D  The pleuroperitoneal membranes, produced as the lungs and pleural cavities expand by invading the body walls, form caudal partitions in the pericardioperitoneal canals.  These membranes gradually grow medially and fuse during the sixth week with the dorsal mesentery of the esophagus and the septum transversum to form the diaphragm.  Failure of one of these membranes to form results in a congenital diaphragmatic hernia through which the abdominal viscera can herniate.  The defect usually appears in the region of the left kidney.

23. C  The epithelium and the glands of the esophagus are derived from the foregut.  The muscular and fibrous elements of the esophagus are derived from the surrounding splanchnic mesenchyme.  The foregut also gives rise to the epithelium and the glands of the lower respiratory tract.  Faulty partitioning of the foregut into the esophagus and trachea during the fourth and fifth weeks results in a tracheosophageal fistula.

24.    E  The esophageal mesentery (dorsal mesentery of the esophagus) is one of the components of the primitive diaphragm.  The other components are the septum transversum and the pleuroperitoneal membranes.  Later a fourth component, the body wall, contributes to peripheral regions of the diaphragm.  The esophageal mesentery constitutes the median portion of the diaphragm.  The crura of the diaphragm develop from muscle fibers which form in the dorsal mesentery of the esophagus.

25.    A  The pericardioperitoneal canals become the pleural cavities.  The lung buds grow laterally during the fifth week and evaginate (push into) the medial walls of the canals.  The inner walls of the canals become the visceral pleura and the outer walls become the parietal pleura.

26.    B  The septum transversum gives rise to the central tendon of the diaphragm.  It is a thick mass of mesenchyme located caudal to the heart.  While located opposite the cervical region of the spinal cord, the septum transversum is invaded by developing muscle tissue from the third, fourth, and fifth myotome regions of the cervical somites.  Later the diaphragm descends until its dorsal part lies at the level of the first lumbar vertebra.  Thus, the seemingly curious origin and course of the phrenic nerves results from the developmental origin of the septum transversum.

---

NOTES:

# THE BRANCHIAL APPARATUS AND THE HEAD AND NECK

O B J E C T I V E S

BE ABLE TO
_____

o    Explain what is meant by the term 'branchial apparatus'.
o    List and illustrate the components of the branchial arches.
o    Construct and label diagrams showing the derivatives of the bran-
     chial arch cartilages.
o    Discuss the formation of the pharyngeal pouches, indicating their
     adult derivatives.
o    Describe the development of the tongue and thyroid gland.
o    Discuss the embryological basis of: ectopic thyroid gland,
     thyroglossal duct cysts and sinuses.
o    Illustrate the development of the face and palate, describing the
     embryological basis of cleft lip and cleft palate.
o    Write brief notes on: branchial cysts, sinuses, and fistulas; the
     first arch syndrome and the DiGeorge syndrome.

_____


F I V E - C H O I C E   C O M P L E T I O N   Q U E S T I O N S


DIRECTIONS:  Each of the following statements or questions is followed by five
suggested responses or completions.  SELECT THE ONE BEST ANSWER in each case and
then circle the appropriate letter at the right of each question.


1.  The branchial apparatus is composed of

    A.  branchial grooves          D.  branchial membranes
    B.  branchial arches           E.  all of the above
    C.  pharyngeal pouches                               A B C D E

2.  The third branchial arch cartilage gives rise to which of the
    following structures?

    A.  Stylohyoid ligament        D.  Sphenomandibular ligament
    B.  Thyroid cartilage          E.  Greater cornu of the
    C.  Styloid process                hyoid bone              A B C D E

<u>SELECT THE ONE BEST ANSWER</u>

3. Which of the following structures is <u>not</u> related to the first branchial arch?

    A. Malleus
    B. Facial nerve
    C. Meckel's cartilage

    D. Mandibular prominence
    E. Maxillary prominence

    A B C D E

4. Which of the following structures is <u>not</u> derived from the second (branchial) arch cartilage?

    A. Incus
    B. Stapes
    C. Styloid process
    D. Lesser cornu of the hyoid bone
    E. Superior part of the hyoid bone

    A B C D E

5. Branchial arches are first recognizable around the middle of the ____ week of development.

    A. third
    B. fourth
    C. fifth

    D. sixth
    E. none of the above

    A B C D E

6. The cartilages of the larynx are derived mainly from the cartilages of which of the following arches?

    A. Second and third
    B. Third and fourth
    C. Third, fourth, and fifth

    D. Fourth and sixth
    E. Fourth and fifth

    A B C D E

7. Muscle elements in the second pair of branchial arches give rise to which of the following muscles?

    A. Frontalis
    B. Platysma
    C. Orbicularis oculi

    D. Buccinator
    E. All of the above

    A B C D E

8. Which of the following cranial nerves supplies muscles derived from the first pair of branchial arches?

    A. Vagus
    B. Glossopharyngeal
    C. Facial

    D. Trigeminal
    E. None of the above

    A B C D E

9. How many <u>well-defined</u> pairs of human pharyngeal pouches develop?

    A. 2
    B. 3
    C. 4

    D. 5
    E. 6

    A B C D E

SELECT THE ONE BEST ANSWER

10. Structures derived from the first pharyngeal pouch include:

    A. tympanic antrum            D. auditory tube
    B. tympanic cavity            E. all of the above
    C. tubotympanic recess                              A B C D E

11. The most common congenital malformation of the head and neck is

    A. cleft palate               D. unilateral cleft lip
    B. bilateral cleft lip        E. median cleft lip
    C. oblique facial cleft                             A B C D E

12. Which of the following structures is derived from the fourth
    pair of pharyngeal pouches?

    A. Thymic corpuscles          D. Thymus gland
    B. Superior parathyroid glands E. All of the above
    C. Inferior parathyroid glands                      A B C D E

13. A young infant had a small blind pit on the side of the neck
    along the anterior border of the sternocleidomastoid muscle.
    Intermittently mucus dripped from its opening. What is the
    most likely embryological basis of this congenital malforma-
    tion of the neck? Persistence of the embryonic opening of the

    A. second pharyngeal pouch    D. thyroglossal duct
    B. second pouch and groove    E. second groove and
    C. third branchial groove        cervical sinus        A B C D E

14. Cleft lip, with or without cleft palate, occurs about once
    in 900 births. Which of the following is considered to be
    an important causative factor in the production of this mal-
    formation?

    A. Riboflavin deficiency      D. Cortisone
    B. Infectious disease         E. Irradiation
    C. Mutant genes                                     A B C D E

15. The major portion of the human palate develops from the

    A. lateral palatine processes  D. medial nasal prominences
    B. median palatine process     E. frontonasal elevation
    C. intermaxillary segment                          A B C D E

======================= ANSWERS, NOTES, AND EXPLANATIONS =========================

1. E  Branchial arches, branchial grooves (clefts), branchial membranes, and

107

pharyngeal pouches of the cranial end of the foregut (primitive pharynx) are parts of the human branchial apparatus which develops during the fourth week of development. The branchial apparatus is subsequently transformed into various structures in the head and neck. For example, the pharyngeal pouches become modified to form structures like the tympanic cavity and the parathyroid and thymus glands.

2. E The cartilages of the third pair of branchial arches give rise to the greater cornua of the hyoid bone, and to the inferior part of the body of this bone. The lesser cornua and the superior part of the body of the hyoid bone are derived from the second branchial arch cartilages.

3. B The facial nerve is not a component of the first or mandibular arch; it is the nerve of the second or hyoid arch. The nerve of the first or mandibular arch is in the trigeminal (CNV). The malleus is derived from the dorsal end of the first arch cartilage. The mandibular prominence is the larger of the two prominences of the first arch; it forms one side of the mandible. The maxillary prominence of the first arch, smaller than the mandibular prominence, contributes to the maxilla. Meckel's cartilage is the name often given to the first arch cartilage; it gives rise to two middle ear bones (malleus and incus), but the mandible forms by intramembranous bone formation around Meckel's cartilage as it degenerates.

4. A The incus is not derived from the second branchial arch cartilage. It is formed by endochondral ossification of the dorsal end of the first arch cartilage (Meckel's cartilage). In addition to the derivatives of the second arch cartilage listed, the stylohyoid ligament is derived from its perichondrium.

5. B The first and second pairs of branchial arches are visible on each side of the future head and neck region by about 24 days. The third pair is recognizable by 26 days, and four pairs are present by the end of the fourth week. The fifth and sixth pairs of arches are rudimentary and are not recognizable externally. As the branchial arches form, the endoderm of the primitive pharynx bulges outward between adjacent arches to form the pharyngeal pouches.

6. D The thyroid, cricoid, arytenoid, corniculate, and cuneiform cartilages are derived mainly from the fused cartilages of the fourth and sixth arch cartilages. The fifth branchial arch is rudimentary and soon degenerates; often it does not develop. The cartilage in the epiglottis develops later than the other cartilages from mesenchyme derived from the hypobranchial eminence, a derivative of the third and fourth pair of branchial arches.

7. E All these muscles are derived from myoblasts that differentiate from mesenchyme in the second pair of branchial arches. During development, some myoblasts from the second branchial arch migrate into the head, mainly to the facial region, and give rise to the muscles of facial expression. During their extensive migration, the developing muscles take their nerve supply (the facial nerve) with them from the second branchial arch.

8. D The fifth cranial nerve (trigeminal nerve) supplies the muscles of mastication and other muscles derived from myoblasts in the first branchial arch.

Because it supplies branchial muscles, the trigeminal nerve and other branchial arch nerves are classified as branchial nerves. Because mesenchyme from the branchial arches also contributes to the dermis and mucous membranes of the head and neck, these areas are supplied with sensory or branchial afferent fibers in the same nerve. The ophthalmic division of the trigeminal nerve does not supply any branchial arch derivatives.

9. C There are four well-defined pairs of pharyngeal pouches. The fifth pair is rudimentary or does not form. If present, they either disappear or are incorporated into the fourth pharyngeal pair of pouches to form the so-called caudal pharyngeal complex.

10. E All these structures are derived from the first pharyngeal pouch. It expands into an elongate, tubotympanic recess which envelops the middle ear bones (auditory ossicles) derived from the dorsal ends of the first and second branchial arch cartilages. The stalk of the tubotympanic recess gives rise to the lining of the auditory tube, and the expanded distal part becomes the lining of the tympanic cavity and antrum of the middle ear.

11. D Cleft lip, with or without cleft palate, occurs about once in 900 births. Unilateral cleft lip is more common than bilateral cleft lip. Cleft palate, with or without cleft lip, occurs about once in 2500 births. Median cleft lip and oblique facial clefts are very uncommon congenital malformations. It must be appreciated that cleft lip and cleft palate are embryologically and etiologically distinct malformations.

12. B The superior parathyroid glands are derived from the fourth pair of pharyngeal pouches. All the other structures are derived from the third pair of pouches. One would think the superior parathyroid glands would be derived from the third rather than the fourth pair of pouches. The reason they are not is that the parathyroids from the third pair of pharyngeal pouches are attached to the thymus gland and descend with it to a more inferior level than the parathyroids derived from the fourth pair of pouches.

13. E Most likely the malformation is an external branchial or lateral cervical sinus, resulting from the persistence of the opening into the cervical sinus. During the fifth week, the second branchial (hyoid) arch grows over the third and fourth arches, forming an ectodermal depression known as the cervical sinus. Normally the second branchial groove and the opening into the cervical sinus are obliterated as the neck forms. If the opening persists, it usually appears as an external opening on the side of the inferior third of the neck. If the second pharyngeal pouch and branchial groove persisted (choice B), a branchial fistula would form and open on the neck, but these are not so common as branchial sinuses. Thyroglossal duct sinuses, formed following infection of a thyroglossal duct cyst, usually open in the midline of the neck anterior to the laryngeal cartilages.

14. C Cleft lip in animals appears to have a mixed genetic and environmental causation, but practically nothing is known at present about environmental factors that may be involved in the production of the malformation in human embryos. A riboflavin deficient diet given to pregnant rats will produce

cleft lip in the fetuses, but is not known to be a causative factor in humans. Experimental work in mice has consistently shown that cortisone causes cleft palate in a high incidence of fetuses, but it is not known to cause cleft lip in mouse or human embryos. Studies in humans indicate that genetic factors are of more importance in cleft lip, with or without cleft palate, than in cleft palate alone. If the parents are normal and have one child with a cleft lip, the chance that the next child will have a cleft lip is four percent. If, however, one of the parents has a cleft lip and they have a child with a cleft lip, the probability that the next child will be affected is 17 percent. Thus, mutant genes appear to be the most important causative factors.

15. A  The lateral palatine processes of the maxillary prominences of the first pair of branchial arches give rise to the posterior or secondary palate. The primary palate or median palatine process develops from the innermost portion of the intermaxillary segment of the upper jaw. This segment, derived from the merged medial nasal prominences, gives rise to the small premaxillary region of the palate.


# M U L T I - C O M P L E T I O N   Q U E S T I O N S


DIRECTIONS:  In each of the following questions or incomplete statements ONE OR MORE of the completions is correct. At the lower right of each question, circle A if 1, 2, and 3 are correct; B if 1 and 3 are correct; C if 2 and 4 are correct; D if only 4 is correct; and E if all are correct.


1.  Structures derived from the first branchial arch include:

    1. malleus
    2. stapes
    3. masseter muscle
    4. stylohyoid ligament                                    A B C D E

2.  Structures derived from endoderm of the second pharyngeal pouch include:

    1. thymus gland
    2. lymph nodules
    3. inferior parathyroid gland
    4. epithelium of the palatine tonsil                      A B C D E

3.  Structures derived from the fourth pair of pharyngeal pouches include:

    1. corpuscles of the thymus gland
    2. superior parathyroid gland
    3. small lymphocytes or thymocytes
    4. parafollicular cells of the thyroid gland              A B C D E

| A | B | C | D | E |
|---|---|---|---|---|
| 1,2,3 | 1,3 | 2,4 | only 4 | all correct |

4. The thyroid gland begins to develop around the middle
of the fourth week

   1. caudal to the median tongue bud
   2. as a median endodermal thickening
   3. in the floor of the primitive pharynx
   4. as a derivative of the third pharyngeal pouch      A B C D E

5. The foramen cecum of the tongue

   1. is a groove separating the body and root of the tongue
   2. is a vestigial, blind pit in the dorsum of the tongue
   3. indicates the line of fusion of the parts of the tongue
   4. indicates the former opening of the thyroglossal duct      A B C D E

6. Structures that make a major contribution to the formation
of the anterior two-thirds of the adult tongue include:

   1. mandibular arches
   2. median tongue bud
   3. distal tongue buds
   4. copula      A B C D E

7. The face of a newborn infant is small because of the

   1. small size of the maxillary sinuses
   2. small size of the nasal cavities
   3. unerupted primary teeth
   4. rudimentary jaws      A B C D E

8. The lateral palatine processes of the maxillary prominences

   1. gradually grow medially and fuse in the midline
   2. begin to fuse anteriorly during the ninth week
   3. fuse with the primary palate and the nasal septum
   4. are completely fused posteriorly by the tenth week      A B C D E

9. Unilateral cleft lip results from

   1. failure of the maxillary prominence on the affected
      side to merge with the intermaxillary segment
   2. breakdown of the epithelium and other tissues in the
      floor of the persistent labial groove
   3. failure of the mesenchyme in the intermaxillary segment
      and the maxillary prominence to proliferate normally
   4. failure of mergence of the maxillary prominence with
      the lateral nasal prominence on the affected side      A B C D E

| A | B | C | D | E |
|---|---|---|---|---|
| 1,2,3 | 1,3 | 2,4 | only 4 | all correct |

10. A unilateral cleft of the posterior palate results from failure of the lateral palatine process on the affected side to fuse with the

    1. median palatine process
    2. nasal septum
    3. mesenchyme in the primitive palate
    4. other lateral palatine process          A B C D E

11. The frontonasal prominence gives rise to the

    1. forehead
    2. sides of the face
    3. dorsum of the nose
    4. sides of the nose          A B C D E

12. Musculature of the human tongue is generally believed to be derived from myoblasts that

    1. migrate from the lateral mesoderm
    2. are derived from the first and third branchial arches
    3. are derived from mesenchyme located ventral to the brain
    4. migrate from the myotome regions of the occipital somites          A B C D E

13. Abnormal transformation of first branchial arch components into their adult derivatives may give rise to which of the following congenital malformations?

    1. Hypoplasia of the mandible
    2. Abnormalities of the ossicles
    3. Deformed external ear
    4. Fish-mouth deformity          A B C D E

14. A young infant presents with a painless swelling in the median plane of the neck, just inferior to the hyoid bone. The mass moves superiorly when the tongue is protruded or during swallowing. From your embryological knowledge, what would you include in the differential diagnosis?

    1. branchial cyst
    2. thyroglossal cyst
    3. branchial vestige
    4. ectopic thyroid gland          A B C D E

| A | B | C | D | E |
|---|---|---|---|---|
| 1,2,3 | 1,3 | 2,4 | only 4 | all correct |

15. An infant had no thymus or parathyroid glands (DiGeorge
    syndrome), and showed hypoparathyroidism. Other malfor-
    mations present were: fish mouth deformity, low-set
    notched ears, and cardiac defects. The embryological
    basis of the thymic aplasia and the absence of the para-
    thyroid glands would be failure of differentiation of the:

    1. dorsal portions of the third pair of pharyngeal pouches
    2. ventral portions of the third pair of pharyngeal pouches
    3. dorsal portions of the fourth pair of pharyngeal pouches
    4. ventral portions of the fourth pair of pharyngeal pouches    A B C D E


======================= ANSWERS, NOTES, AND EXPLANATIONS =========================

1. B  1 and 3 are correct.  The malleus, a middle ear bone, develops by endochondral ossification of the dorsal end of the first branchial arch cartilage
   (Meckel's cartilage).  The masseter, one of the muscles of mastication, develops from myoblasts derived from mesenchyme in the first branchial arch.
   This first arch forms four of the five primordia of the face (the other is
   the frontonasal prominence).  All muscles of mastication are derived from
   myoblasts in the first branchial or mandibular arch.  The stapes and
   stylohyoid ligament are derived from the cartilage of the second branchial or
   hyoid arch.

2. D  4 only is correct.  The endoderm of the second pharyngeal pouch gives rise
   to the surface epithelium and the lining of the crypts of the palatine
   tonsils.  The lymphoid tissue of the lymph nodules is derived from the
   mesenchyme around the pouch.  The thymus gland and the inferior parathyroid
   glands are derived from the third pair of pharyngeal pouches.

3. C  2 and 4 are correct.  The superior parathyroid glands are derived from the
   fourth pair of pharyngeal pouches.  The thymus and the corpuscles or bodies
   of the thymus are derived from the third pharyngeal pouches.  The ultimobranchial bodies are derived mainly from the fourth pair of pouches.  They
   may receive contributions from the fifth pouches.  These bodies become
   incorporated into the thyroid gland and disseminate to form the
   parafollicular or C cells which produce calcitonin.

4. A  1, 2, and 3 are correct.  The thyroid is the first endocrine gland to
   begin developing.  It appears on about day 24 as a thickening in the
   endodermal floor of the primitive pharynx (cranial end of the foregut).  It
   develops just caudal to the median tongue bud (tuberculum impar).  It is not
   derived from any of the pharyngeal pouches.

5. C  2 and 4 are correct.  The foramen cecum is a median pit on the dorsum of

113

the posterior part of the tongue. It was the site of origin of the thyroid gland in the embryo. From it, the limbs of the V-shaped terminal sulcus run rostrally and laterally. It is a nonfunctional structure that persists in the tongue after the thyroglossal duct disappears. If the thyroglossal duct persists, the foramen cecum forms the opening of an internal thyroglossal duct sinus.

6.  B  1 and 3 are correct.  The anterior two-thirds of the tongue or body is derived from the distal tongue buds. These swellings or elevations result from proliferation of mesenchyme in the ventromedial portions of the first pair of branchial arches. The median tongue bud and the copula make no significant contribution to the adult tongue.

7.  E  All are correct.  All these factors cause the face to be small in the new-born. Eruption of the primary teeth usually occurs between the sixth and twenty-fourth month after birth. The nasal cavities and paranasal sinuses expand during infancy and childhood. The sinuses extend into the maxilla, ethmoid, frontal, and sphenoid bones. They do not reach their maximum size until around puberty. The jaws develop as the deciduous teeth erupt and the permanent teeth develop. During the fourth year, well developed deciduous and permanent teeth are present in the jaws, but the permanent teeth do not begin to erupt until the seventh year.

8.  A  1, 2, and 3 are correct.  The fusion of the lateral palatine processes is not complete until the end of the twelfth week. This is important to remember because environmental agents might affect fusion of the processes during the early part of the fetal period, causing clefts of the posterior palate. It is well established that cortisone will cause cleft palate in a high incidence of newborn mice and rabbits if given to their mothers at the critical period of development of the palate. There is no conclusive evidence to indicate that cortisone causes cleft palate or any other human malformation.

9.  A  1, 2, and 3 are correct.  Unilateral cleft lip is the most common of all facial malformations. It occurs about once in 900 births and is more common than bilateral or median cleft lip. Cleft lip occurs more often on the left than the right side, and the incidence is higher in males. Most cases have a multifactorial origin, but some cases are associated with single, mutant genes. In unilateral cleft lip, there is failure of the maxillary prominence on the affected side to merge with the merged medial nasal prominences (intermaxillary segment). Failure of mergence of the maxillary prominence with the lateral nasal prominence (choice 4), would result in an orbitofacial cleft.

10.  C  2 and 4 are correct.  Unilateral cleft of the posterior palate results when there is a failure of mesenchymal proliferation in the lateral palatine process of the maxillary prominence of the first branchial arch. As a result, the process does not grow medially and fuse with the other lateral palatine process and the nasal septum. The lateral palatine process fuses with the median palatine process (primitive palate). However, if failure of these processes to fuse also occurs, a unilateral cleft of the anterior and posterior palates results, i.e., a complete cleft palate.

11.  B  1 and 3 are correct.  The superior parts of the face are mainly derived from the maxillary prominences of the first branchial arch.  The rest of the superior facial region, i.e., the dorsum of the nose and the forehead, is derived from the frontonasal prominence.  The alae or sides of the nose are derived from the lateral nasal prominences.

12.  C  2 and 4 are correct.  In submammalian forms, there is no doubt that the tongue musculature arises by migration of myoblasts from the occipital somites, accompanied by the XII cranial nerve.  The evidence for this migration in human embryos is not conclusive.  It is reasonable to assume that this migration of myoblasts occurs because the tongue muscle is supplied by the hypoglossal nerve.  There is also general agreement that some of the myoblasts that form tongue muscles probably differentiate from mesenchymal cells derived from mesoderm in the first and third branchial arches.  Although initially involved in tongue development, mesenchyme from the second branchial arches is soon overgrown by third arch mesenchyme.

13.  A  1, 2, and 3 are correct.  These malformations and others are commonly associated with two rare symptom complexes: (1) Treacher-Collins syndrome (mandibulofacial dysostosis); and (2) Pierre Robin syndrome.  The initiating cause of the Pierre Robin syndrome appears to be poor development of the mandibular area, allowing the tongue to be located more posteriorly than normal.  As a result, the palatine processes do not fuse.  Maldevelopment of the ears is understandable in view of their association in development with the first arch.  The fish-mouth deformity is often associated with DiGeorge syndrome caused by failure of the third and fourth pharyngeal pouches to differentiate normally.

14.  C  2 and 4 are correct.  A thyroglossal cyst is the most likely diagnosis.  These remnants of the thyroglossal duct may be located anywhere from the base of the tongue, near the foramen cecum, to the isthmus of the thyroid gland.  This is the course followed by this gland during its descent through the neck.  Remnants of the duct, usually in the region of the hyoid bone, may form cysts.  Because the cell rest that gives rise to the cyst is present at birth, thyroglossal duct cysts are classified as congenital malformations.  A midline swelling in the neck could also be caused by an ectopic thyroid (cervical thyroid), but this is an uncommon condition.  In these cases, the thyroid gland does not descend to its usual site in front of the trachea.  Branchial cysts and vestiges are usually found in the side of the neck, anterior to the sternocleidomastoid muscle.

15.  A  1, 2, and 3 are correct.  The inferior parathyroid glands differentiate from the dorsal portions of the third pair of pharyngeal pouches.  The thymus gland forms from the ventral portions of the third pair of pharyngeal pouches while ventral portions of the fourth pair rise to the ultimobranchial bodies which disseminate to form the parafollicular cells of the thyroid gland.  The fish-mouth deformity and the abnormal ears suggest that there was also maldevelopment of the first branchial arch.  There is no apparent genetic basis for DiGeorge syndrome.  The malformations could result from teratogens interfering with the transformation of the branchial apparatus into its adult derivatives.

# F I V E - C H O I C E   A S S O C I A T I O N   Q U E S T I O N S

DIRECTIONS: Each group of questions below consists of a numbered list of descriptive words or phrases accompanied by a diagram with certain parts indicated by letters, or by a list of lettered headings. For each numbered word or phrase, SELECT THE LETTERED PART OR HEADING that matches it correctly. Then insert the letter in the space to the right of the appropriate number. Sometimes more than one numbered word or phrase may be correctly matched to the same lettered part or heading.

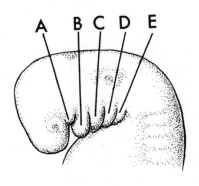

1. _____ Supplied by the vagus nerve
2. _____ Its cartilage forms the stapes
3. _____ Forms inferior part of the face
4. _____ Gives rise to the lateral palatine process
5. _____ Its muscle element gives rise to the platysma
6. _____ Its cartilage forms a greater cornu of the hyoid bone

A. First branchial arch
B. Second branchial arch
C. Third branchial arch

D. Fourth branchial arch
E. Sixth branchial arch

7. _____ Glossopharyngeal nerve
8. _____ Muscles of facial expression
9. _____ Supplied by the maxillary division of the fifth cranial nerve
10. _____ Stylohyoid ligament
11. _____ Superior laryngeal branch of the vagus nerve
12. _____ Meckel's cartilage
13. _____ Gives rise to the lateral palatine process
14. _____ Greater cornua of the hyoid bone
15. _____ Forms lateral part of the upper lip
16. _____ Lesser cornua of the hyoid bone
17. _____ A main contributor of the thyroid cartilage
18. _____ Supplied by CN X

## ASSOCIATION QUESTIONS

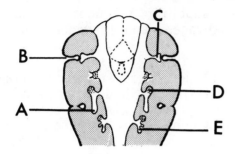

19. _____ Becomes the external acoustic meatus
20. _____ Becomes the inferior para-thyroid gland
21. _____ Tubotympanic recess
22. _____ Gives rise to the ultimobran-chial body
23. _____ Forms half of the thymus gland
24. _____ Gives rise to the auditory tube

A. First pharyngeal pouch
B. Second pharnygeal pouch
C. Third pharyngeal pouch

D. Fourth pharyngeal pouch
E. Fifth pharnygeal pouch

25. _____ Thymus gland
26. _____ Superior parathyroid gland
27. _____ Inferior parathyroid gland
28. _____ May not develop

29. _____ Palatine tonsil
30. _____ Tubotympanic recess
31. _____ Internal branchial sinus
32. _____ Thyrocalcitonin

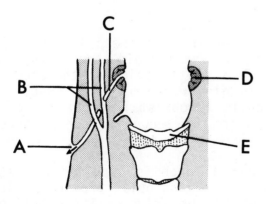

33. _____ Derived from the second and third branchial arch cartilages
34. _____ Internal branchial sinus
35. _____ Derived from the second branch-ial groove and cervical sinus
36. _____ External branchial sinus
37. _____ Internal and external carotid arteries
38. _____ Organ derived from the second pharyngeal pouch and mesenchyme

==================== ANSWERS, NOTES, AND EXPLANATIONS ========================

1. E  The fourth branchial arch is supplied by the superior laryngeal branch of the vagus nerve (CN X).  This nerve supplies pharyngeal and laryngeal muscles that develop from the fourth branchial arch.

2. C  The dorsal end of the second arch cartilage (Reichert's cartilage) ossifies to form the stapes of the middle ear and the styloid process of the temporal bone.  The ventral ends of the cartilages give rise to the lesser cornua and superior part of the body of the hyoid bone.  The perichondrium of this cartilage forms the stylohyoid ligament.

3. B  The mandibular prominences of the first branchial arches form the inferior part of the face.  The mandible develops in these prominences by intramembranous bone formation around the first arch cartilages.  The superior part of the face forms from the maxillary prominences of the first branchial arches.

4. A  The lateral palatine processes arise as horizontal mesenchymal projections from the inner surfaces of the maxillary prominences of the first branchial arches.  The lateral palatine processes grow toward each other and fuse.

5. C  The muscle elements in the second branchial arches give rise to myoblasts which migrate into the facial region and around the ears and the eyes.  These myoblasts differentiate into the muscles of facial expression.

6. D  The third arch cartilages, located in the ventral portions of the arches, ossify to form the greater cornua and the inferior part of the body of the hyoid bone.

7. C  The glossopharyngeal nerve (CN IX) is the nerve of the third branchial arch; hence it supplies the stylopharyngeus muscle derived from the muscle element in this arch.  As the dorsal part of the root of the tongue is derived from the third arch, its sensory innervation is partly supplied by the glossopharyngeal nerve.

8. B  The muscles of facial expression are derived from the second branchial arch.  Other muscles derived from this arch are the stylohyoid, the posterior belly of the digastric, and the stapedius.  From the position of the second arch in the embryo, one would not expect it to give rise to facial muscles.  During development, the developing muscle cells (myoblasts) migrate to the head and retain their original nerve supply from the second branchial arch (i.e., the facial nerve).

9. A  The maxillary prominence of the first branchial arch is supplied by the maxillary division of the trigeminal (CN V).  The mandibular prominence is supplied by the mandibular branch of this nerve.  The trigeminal nerve also supplies the muscles of mastication and other muscles derived from this arch.

This nerve also supplies the skin over the mandible and the anterior two-thirds of the tongue.

10. B  The stylohyoid ligament is derived from the perichondrium of the second branchial arch cartilage, after it regresses between the styloid process and the hyoid bone.

11. D  The superior laryngeal branch of the vagus (CN X) supplies the fourth branchial arch. Hence, it supplies the cricothyroid muscle and the constrictors of the pharynx that are derived from the muscle element in this arch.

12. B  Meckel's cartilage is the name often given to the cartilage located in the mandibular process of the first branchial arch. Its dorsal portion, related to the developing internal ear, becomes ossified to form two middle ear bones (malleus and incus).

13. A  The internal parts of the maxillary prominences of the first pair of branchial arches give rise to two horizontal projections called lateral palatine processes. These processes later fuse with each other and with the nasal septum to form the posterior or secondary palate. Incomplete fusion of these processes results in a cleft of the posterior palate.

14. D  The greater cornua of the hyoid bone are derived from the cartilages of the third pair of branchial arches. The inferior part of the body of this bone is also derived by endochondral ossification of the cartilages of these arches.

15. A  The maxillary prominence of the first branchial arch gives rise to the lateral part of the upper lip. It fuses with the intermaxillary segment (merged medial nasal prominences) which gives rise to the central portion or philtrum of the lip.

16. C  The lesser cornua of the hyoid bone are derived from the cartilages of the second branchial arches. The superior part of the body of this bone is also derived by endochondral ossification of these cartilages.

17. E  The cartilaginous components of the fourth pair of branchial arches give rise to large parts of the thyroid cartilage. The cartilages of the sixth arches are also main contributors.

18. E  The fourth branchial arch is supplied by the vagus nerve (CN X). This nerve supplies the intrinsic muscles of the larynx which develop from myoblasts in the fourth branchial arch.

19. B  The external acoustic meatus develops from the dorsal end of the first branchial groove. All other branchial grooves normally disappear as the neck forms.

20. D  The solid dorsal bulbar portion of the third pharyngeal pouch differentiates into an inferior parathyroid gland. These glands descend with

the thymus gland and later leave it to lie on the posterior surface of the thyroid gland.

21.　C　The tubotympanic recess gives rise to the auditory tube, the tympanic cavity and antrum. Its epithelium gives rise to the internal layer of the tympanic membrane.

22.　E　The ventral portions of the fourth pair of pharyngeal pouches give rise to the ultimobranchial bodies. If present, the fifth pair of pouches may also contribute to the formation of these bodies. The ultimobranchial bodies later fuse with the thyroid gland and are represented by cells called light or parafollicular cells. These cells produce calcitonin, an important hormone concerned with calcium metabolism.

23.　A　The ventral portions of the third pair of pharyngeal pouches fuse and give rise to the primordium of the thymus gland. This thymic mass becomes invaded by mesenchymal cells that break up the gland into lobules. The thymic corpuscles (Hassall's corpuscles) appear to be derived from the endodermal epithelium. The origin of the thymocytes is controversial, but they are generally believed to be mesenchymal in origin.

24.　C　The tubotympanic recess gives rise to the epithelium and glands of the auditory tube. The bony wall in its posterior third and the remaining cartilaginous wall are derived from the surrounding mesenchyme.

25.　C　The elongate ventral portions of the third pair of pharyngeal pouches migrate medially and fuse to form the primordium of the thymus gland. Development of the thymus is not complete at birth; it continues to grow and reaches its greatest size at puberty. Thereafter it becomes smaller.

26.　D　The dorsal bulbar portion of each fourth pharyngeal pouch develops into a superior parathyroid gland. They come to lie on the dorsal surface of the thyroid gland.

27.　C　The dorsal bulbar portion of each third pharyngeal pouch differentiates into a parathyroid gland. These glands migrate caudally with the thymus gland which develops from the ventral portions of this pair of pouches. Hence, the parathyroid glands derived from the third pair of pouches come to lie further caudally than those from the fourth pair of pouches. Because of this descent, the inferior parathyroid glands are sometimes located in other than their normal position, i.e., they may be drawn into the thorax by the descent of the thymus.

28.　E　The fifth pair of pharyngeal pouches often do not develop. When present, they are rudimentary and are incorporated into the fourth pair of pharyngeal pouches.

29.　B　The palatine tonsils are derived from the endoderm of the second pair of pharyngeal pouches and the associated mesenchyme. The endoderm of the pouches gives rise to the surface epithelium and the lining of the crypts of the tonsil. The mesenchyme around the developing crypts differentiates into lymphoid tissue.

30.  A  The epithelium and the glands of the auditory tube are derived from the elongate tubotympanic recess, the expanded first pharyngeal pouch. This recess also gives rise to the tympanic cavity and antrum. The connective tissue and cartilaginous parts of the auditory tube are derived from the mesenchyme surrounding the tubotympanic recess.

31.  B  Internal branchial sinuses open into the pharynx. Usually they are derived from a remnant of the second pharyngeal pouch; hence they often open into the intratonsillar cleft, the remains of the opening into the second pharyngeal pouch.

32.  D  Calcitonin is produced by the parafollicular cells (C cells) of the thyroid gland, derived from the ultimobranchial bodies. These bodies develop from the ventral portions of the fourth pair of pharyngeal pouches. If the fifth pair of pouches develops, they may contribute to the formation of the ultimobranchial bodies.

33.  E  The hyoid bone develops by endochondral ossification of the ventral ends of the second and third branchial arch cartilages. The second arch cartilages give rise to the lesser cornua and the superior part of the body, and the third arch cartilages give rise to the greater cornua and the inferior part of the body of the hyoid bone.

34.  C  Internal branchial sinuses opening into the pharynx are very rare. Because they almost always open into the intratonsillar cleft or near the palatopharyngeal arch, these sinuses usually result from partial persistence of part of the second pharyngeal pouch. Usually these pouches give rise to to the epithelium and the lining of the crypts of the palatine tonsils.

35.  A  External branchial sinuses (also called lateral cervical sinuses) are uncommon. Almost all those that open on the side of the neck result from failure of the second branchial groove to obliterate. The sinuses usually open on the inferior one-third of a line that runs from the auricle along the anterior border of the sternocleidomastoid muscle to the jugular notch. Often there is an intermittent discharge of mucus from the opening, resulting from infection of the sinus.

36.  A  External branchial (lateral cervical) sinuses are lined with stratified squamous or columnar epithelium; they are surrounded by a muscular wall. Thus, by pulling the skin inferiorly, it is possible to palpate the firm sinus as it extends superiorly.

37.  B  Sinuses and fistulas ascend through the subcutaneous tissue, the platysma muscle, and between the external and internal carotid arteries.

38.  D  The surface epithelium and the lining of the crypts of the palatine tonsils are derived from the endoderm of the second pair of pharyngeal pouches. The mesenchyme surrounding the pouches differentiates into lymphoid

tissue which soon becomes organized into lymph nodules.

---

NOTES:

# THE RESPIRATORY SYSTEM

## O B J E C T I V E S

BE ABLE TO:

_____

o   Describe the early development of the lower respiratory system, illustrating the formation of the laryngotracheal tube and its derivatives.

o   List the four stages of lung development and discuss the main events occurring during each period.

o   Write a brief note on surfactant and the respiratory distress syndrome.

o   Discuss and illustrate the embryological basis of tracheoesophageal fistula with esophageal atresia.

_____

## F I V E - C H O I C E   C O M P L E T I O N   Q U E S T I O N S

DIRECTIONS: Each of the following statements or questions is followed by five suggested responses or completions.  SELECT THE ONE BEST ANSWER in each case and then circle the appropriate letter at the right of each question.

1.  The first indication of the lower respiratory tract in the human embryo is the laryngotracheal groove.  It begins to develop in the primitive pharyngeal floor at ____ days.

    A.  19-21            D.  28-30
    B.  22-24            E.  31-33
    C.  25-27                                            A B C D E

2.  The connective tissue, cartilage, and smooth muscle of the trachea are derived from the

    A.  somatic mesoderm from the lateral plates
    B.  splanchnic mesenchyme around the laryngotracheal tube
    C.  endodermal lining of the laryngotracheal tube
    D.  mesenchyme from the fourth to sixth pairs of branchial arches
    E.  neural crest                                     A B C D E

123

SELECT THE ONE BEST ANSWER

3.  One-eighth to one-sixth of the adult number of alveoli are
    present in the lungs at birth.  Their number increases after
    birth for at least ____ years.

    A.  2                        D.  8
    B.  4                        E.  10
    C.  6                                          A B C D E

4.  Each of the following malformations of the lower respiratory
    tract is uncommon except:

    A.  tracheal stenosis        D.  congenital emphysema
    B.  tracheal diverticulum    E.  tracheoesophageal
    C.  tracheal atresia             fistula           A B C D E

5.  Pulmonary surfactant is produced by

    A.  type I alveolar epithelial cells
    B.  blood cells
    C.  alveolar macrophages (phagocytes)
    D.  Endothelial cells
    E.  type II alveolar epithelial cells          A B C D E

6.  Pulmonary surfactant begins to form in the human fetus
    at about ____ weeks.

    A.  16                       D.  28
    B.  20                       E.  32
    C.  24                                         A B C D E

7.  A fetus born prematurely during which of the following
    periods of lung development may survive?

    A.  Organogenetic            D.  Canalicular
    B.  Terminal sac             E.  Embryonic
    C.  Pseudoglandular                            A B C D E

8.  The lungs at birth are about half inflated with liquid
    derived largely from the:

    A.  lung tissues             D.  tracheal glands
    B.  nasal mucus              E.  maternal blood
    C.  amniotic fluid                             A B C D E

======================= ANSWERS, NOTES, AND EXPLANATIONS =========================

1.  C  The median longitudinal laryngotracheal groove is recognizable at about

26 days. As it deepens, its caudal end begins to separate off from the foregut, giving rise to the tracheal and esophageal primordia. This division extends cranially until only the communication between the pharynx and the air passages (the laryngeal aditus) remains.

2. B The connective tissue, cartilage, and smooth muscle of the trachea and bronchi develop from splanchnic mesenchyme around the laryngotracheal tube. The striated muscles, cartilages and connective tissues of the larynx are derived from branchial mesenchyme of the fourth to sixth pairs of branchial arches.

3. D Alveolar production begins in the human lungs during the late fetal period, but characteristic pulmonary alveoli probably do not form until respiration begins. Alveoli continue to form until at least the eighth year. It has been estimated that there are 30-50 million alveoli present at birth and by the eighth year there are about 300 million alveoli present. The number of alveoli in the adult lung varies between 250 and 500 million.

4. E Tracheoesophageal fistula occurs about once in 2500 births, predominantly in males. This connection between the trachea and esophagus results from incomplete separation of the respiratory and digestive portions of the foregut. In most cases, there is also esophageal atresia.

5. E The type II alveolar epithelial cells are believed to produce surfactant, a surface-active agent. Surfactant forms a monomolecular layer over pulmonary alveolar surfaces and is capable of lowering surface tension at the air-alveolar interface when respiration begins at birth, thereby maintaining patency of the alveoli. Absence or deficiency of surfactant is a major cause of hyaline membrane disease.

6. C It is generally agreed that the type II cells of the epithelium of the alveoli, often called secretory cells, begin to produce surfactant at about 24 weeks. It has been suggested that prolonged intrauterine asphyxia may produce reversible changes in these cells, making them incapable of producing surfactant. However, there are likely several causes for absence or deficiency of surfactant, particularly in premature infants.

7. B During the terminal sac period (24 weeks to birth), a fetus may survive if born prematurely, especially if it weighs 1000 or more grams. The terminal air sacs appear as outpouchings of the respiratory bronchioles and are soon surrounded by a rich capillary network. Prior to this time, the fetal lungs are usually incapable of providing adequate gas exchange, mainly because of inadequate pulmonary vasculature.

8. A The fluid in the lungs at birth is believed to be derived mainly from the lower respiratory tract itself. It has been estimated that as much as 30 ml per day of fluid is produced by the fetal tracheobronchial tree near term. The fluid in the lungs differs in composition from plasma, lymph, and amniotic fluid. Some of the liquid in the lungs probably comes from the tracheal glands, and some is likely amniotic fluid. It is well established that respiratory movements occur before birth causing aspiration of amniotic fluid.

## M U L T I - C O M P L E T I O N   Q U E S T I O N S

DIRECTIONS:  In each of the following questions or incomplete statements ONE OR MORE of the completions is correct.  At the lower right of each question, circle A if 1, 2, and 3 are correct; B if 1 and 3 are correct; C if 2 and 4 are correct; D if only 4 is correct; and E if all are correct.

1.  Correct statements about lung development include:

    1.  The laryngotracheal groove develops during the fourth week.
    2.  The laryngotracheal tube is surrounded by splanchnic mesenchyme.
    3.  The laryngotracheal tube gives rise to two bronchial buds.
    4.  The left bronchial bud divides into three buds and the right one divides into two buds.        A B C D E

2.  Correct statements about lung development include:

    1.  Lung development is usually divided into four stages.
    2.  The alveoli have all developed by late infancy.
    3.  By 26 to 28 weeks, the lungs are well enough developed to permit adequate gas exchange.
    4.  Lymphatic capillaries project into the future air spaces.        A B C D E

3.  Developmental periods of the lungs include:

    1.  pseudoglandular
    2.  vascularization
    3.  canalicular
    4.  glandular        A B C D E

4.  Hyaline membrane disease causes respiratory distress and may cause death in newborn infants.  It is

    1.  caused by overdistension of the alveoli
    2.  principally a disease of premature infants
    3.  commonly associated with polyhydramnios
    4.  associated with a deficiency of surfactant        A B C D E

5.  Tracheoesophageal fistula

    1.  is commonly associated with esophageal atresia
    2.  is encountered more often in males than in females
    3.  commonly joins the inferior part of the esophagus to the trachea
    4.  results from unequal partitioning of the foregut into the esophagus and trachea        A B C D E

| A | B | C | D | E |
|---|---|---|---|---|
| 1,2,3 | 1,3 | 2,4 | only 4 | all correct |

6.  The lungs at birth are about half inflated with liquid.
    During and after birth, this fluid is cleared by which
    of the following routes?

    1.  Out of the mouth and nose from the lower airways as
        a result of pressure on the thorax during birth
    2.  Through alveolar and capillary walls into the blood
    3.  Through the alveolar wall into the lymphatics around
        the bronchi and pulmonary vessels
    4.  Into the digestive tract where it is absorbed by the
        intestines and subsequently excreted by the kidneys    A B C D E

7.  A newborn infant coughs and regurgitates its milk when
    fed, and has respiratory distress and abdominal disten-
    tion when it cries.  Congenital malformation(s) that
    you would consider in the differential diagnosis of the
    infant's problems include:

    1.  tracheal atresia
    2.  esophageal atresia
    3.  agenesis of the lungs
    4.  tracheoesophageal fistula    A B C D E

8.  The trachea and bronchi are derived from the

    1.  caudal branchial arch cartilages
    2.  splanchnic mesenchyme
    3.  hypobranchial eminence
    4.  endoderm of the laryngotracheal tube    A B C D E

9.  The larynx is derived from the

    1.  caudal branchial arch cartilages
    2.  endoderm of the laryngotracheal tube
    3.  branchial mesenchyme
    4.  hypobranchial eminence    A B C D E

10. During the canalicular period of lung development, the

    1.  lumina of the bronchi enlarge
    2.  lung tissue becomes vascular
    3.  respiratory bronchioles form
    4.  alveolar epithelium becomes attenuated    A B C D E

11. Tracheoesophageal fistula is often associated with:

    1.  esophageal atresia
    2.  an excess of amniotic fluid
    3.  cyanosis (bluish coloration of the skin)
    4.  incomplete fusion of the laryngeal folds    A B C D E

| A | B | C | D | E |
|---|---|---|---|---|
| 1,2,3 | 1,3 | 2,4 | only 4 | all correct |

12. Concerning lung development, correct statements include:

1. About 1/8 to 1/6 of the adult number of alveoli are present at birth.
2. The adult number of alveoli may be present at birth.
3. The lungs at birth are about half inflated with liquid.
4. By 22 weeks the lungs are usually sufficiently well developed to permit survival of the fetus if born prematurely.

A B C D E

======================== ANSWERS, NOTES, AND EXPLANATIONS ========================

1. A  <u>1, 2, and 3 are correct.</u>  The splanchnic mesenchyme around the laryngotracheal tube gives rise to the connective tissue, cartilage and smooth muscle of the trachea and bronchi.  The mesenchyme forming the connective tissue, cartilages and muscles of the larynx, is derived from the fourth to sixth branchial arches.  The left bronchial bud divides into two buds and the one on the right into three buds.  These divisions establish the primordia of the lobes of the adult lungs.

2. B  <u>1 and 3 are correct.</u>  About one-eighth to one-sixth of the adult number of alveoli are present in a newborn infant.  More develop during infancy, but many alveoli form during childhood.  Lymphatic capillaries develop during the terminal sac period, but they do not project into the alveolar wall.

3. B  <u>1 and 3 are correct.</u>  The terminal sac and alveolar periods follow the two earlier stages mentioned.  Although the lungs initially have a somewhat glandular appearance, no glands form in the lungs.  The type II alveolar cells, however, produce a surface-active agent called surfactant.  Vascularization is an important process during lung development that occurs during all but the pseudoglandular period.

4. C  <u>2 and 4 are correct.</u>  Hyaline membrane disease may occur in a full-term newborn infant, but it occurs most often in premature infants.  Absence or a deficiency of surfactant appears to be a major cause of this disease in which a membrane-like structure lines the respiratory bronchioles, alveolar ducts, and alveoli.  This prevents adequate gas exchange (ventilation of the lungs).

5. A  <u>1, 2, and 3 are correct.</u>  Tracheoesophageal fistula occurs more often in males than females and is commonly associated with atresia of the esophagus.  Gastric secretions are usually aspirated (drawn into the lungs) via the fistula.  This abnormal connection results from incomplete partitioning of the foregut into the esophagus and trachea.  Unequal partitioning would cause tracheal or esophageal stenosis.

6. A <u>1, 2, and 3 are correct</u>. It has been estimated that about one-third of the liquid in the lungs leaves by each of these three routes. Most of the fluid in the fetal lung is thought to be a secretory product of the lung itself. The amount of liquid in the lungs increases during gestation.

7. C <u>2 and 4 are correct</u>. The regurgitation of milk and the coughing suggest esophageal atresia. The food cannot pass into the inferior part of the esophagus and enter the stomach; thus it returns to the pharynx causing coughing and vomiting. The respiratory distress and abdominal distention suggest a tracheoesophageal fistula. Gastric secretions pass from the stomach and enter the trachea via the fistula. Some of this fluid passes out of the airways, but some is aspirated into the lungs. Crying causes an excessive amount of air to enter the stomach and intestines causing abdominal distention. Tracheal atresia and agenesis of the lungs are incompatible with life after birth.

8. C <u>2 and 4 are correct</u>. The endodermal lining of the laryngotracheal tube gives rise to the epithelium of the trachea, bronchi, and lungs and to the bronchotracheal glands. The splanchnic mesenchyme surrounding the tube gives rise to the connective tissue, cartilage, muscle, and to the blood and lymphatic vessels of these structures.

9. A <u>1, 2, and 3 are correct</u>. The epithelium of the larynx is derived from the endoderm of the cranial end of the laryngotracheal tube. Mesenchyme from the fourth to sixth branchial arches gives rise to the connective tissue, cartilages and muscles of the larynx.

10. E <u>All are correct</u>. All these events occur during the canalicular or second period of lung development which extends from 16 weeks to 25 weeks. Although the lungs are rather well developed by the end of this period, fetuses usually die within a few days if born prematurely because the respiratory system is still too immature to provide adequate exchange of gases between the lungs and the blood.

11. A <u>1, 2, and 3 are correct</u>. In the most common type of tracheoesophageal fistula, there is atresia of the esophagus. The superior part of the esophagus ends blindly and the inferior portion joins the trachea near its bifurcation. An excess of amniotic fluid (polyhydramnios) is commonly associated with esophageal atresia because amniotic fluid, normally swallowed by the fetus, cannot pass to the intestines for absorption and subsequent transfer to the placenta for elimination by the mother. Cyanosis (bluish discoloration of skin and mucous membranes) develops within a few hours after birth with the usual type of tracheoesophageal fistula. Cyanosis results from poor oxygenation of the blood caused by the aspiration of gastric contents, mucus, and food. Aspiration of these fluids causes dyspnea (difficult or labored breathing).

12. B <u>1 and 3 are correct</u>. Alveoli form until at least the eighth year. Most of the fluid in the lungs is rapidly replaced with air when respiration begins. Although there is no sharp limit of development, age or weight at which a fetus automatically becomes viable, or beyond which survival is assured, experience has shown that it is unusual for a fetus to survive whose weight is less than 1000 gm or whose fertilization age is less than 26 weeks.

129

# FIVE-CHOICE ASSOCIATION QUESTIONS

DIRECTIONS:  Each group of questions below consists of a numbered list of descriptive words or phrases accompanied by a diagram with certain parts indicated by letters, or by a list of lettered headings.  For each numbered word or phrase, SELECT THE LETTERED PART OR HEADING that matches it correctly.  Then insert the letter in the space to the right of the appropriate number.  Sometimes more than one numbered word or phrase may be correctly matched to the same lettered part or heading.

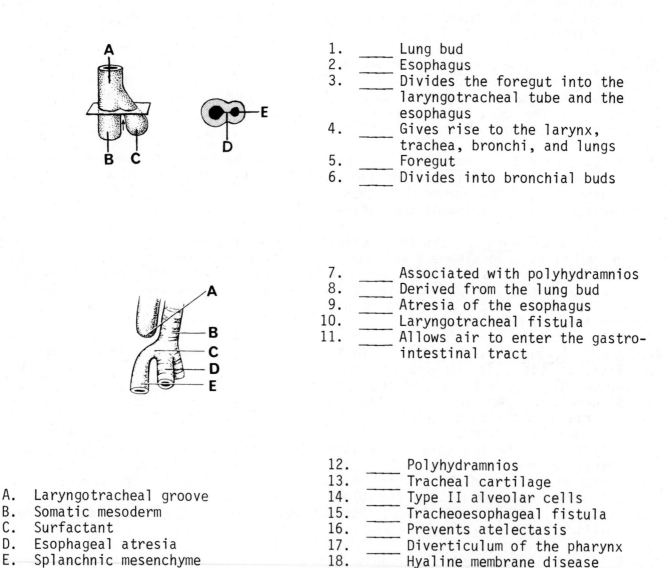

1. _____ Lung bud
2. _____ Esophagus
3. _____ Divides the foregut into the laryngotracheal tube and the esophagus
4. _____ Gives rise to the larynx, trachea, bronchi, and lungs
5. _____ Foregut
6. _____ Divides into bronchial buds

7. _____ Associated with polyhydramnios
8. _____ Derived from the lung bud
9. _____ Atresia of the esophagus
10. _____ Laryngotracheal fistula
11. _____ Allows air to enter the gastro-intestinal tract

A. Laryngotracheal groove
B. Somatic mesoderm
C. Surfactant
D. Esophageal atresia
E. Splanchnic mesenchyme

12. _____ Polyhydramnios
13. _____ Tracheal cartilage
14. _____ Type II alveolar cells
15. _____ Tracheoesophageal fistula
16. _____ Prevents atelectasis
17. _____ Diverticulum of the pharynx
18. _____ Hyaline membrane disease
19. _____ Parietal pleura

## ASSOCIATION QUESTIONS

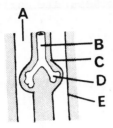

20. _____ Primordium of the left lung
21. _____ Its glands are derived from the laryngotracheal tube
22. _____ Pericardioperitoneal canal
23. _____ Future right pleural cavity
24. _____ Splanchnic mesenchyme
25. _____ Will become the parietal pleura

======================= ANSWERS, NOTES, AND EXPLANATIONS =========================

1.  C  The lung bud develops at the caudal end of the laryngotracheal tube and soon divides into two bronchial buds.  These buds differentiate into the bronchi and their ramifications in the lungs.

2.  B  The esophagus is derived from the foregut and is separated from the laryngotracheal tube by the tracheoesophageal septum.

3.  D  The tracheoesophageal septum, formed by the gradual fusion of the tracheoesophageal folds, divides the foregut into the laryngotracheal tube and the esophagus.  Incomplete separation of these structures results in one of the varieties of tracheoesophageal fistula.

4.  E  The endodermal lining of the laryngotracheal tube gives rise to the epithelium and glands of the larynx, trachea, and bronchi, and to the pulmonary lining epithelium.  The connective tissue, cartilage, and smooth muscle of these structures develop from the surrounding splanchnic mesenchyme.

5.  A  The foregut gives rise to the pharynx and its derivatives, the lower respiratory tract, the esophagus, the stomach, the first part of the duodenum as far as the entry of the bile duct, and to the liver and pancreas.

6.  C  The lung bud that forms at the caudal end of the laryngotracheal tube during the fourth week gives rise to two bronchial buds.  These buds differentiate into the bronchi and their ramifications in the lungs.

7.  A  Polyhydramnios (excess of amniotic fluid) is frequent in mothers of

fetuses that have esophageal atresia because amniotic fluid cannot pass to the intestines for absorption and subsequent transfer to the placenta for transfer. If you selected choice C, you were partly right because esophageal atresia is often associated with tracheoesophageal fistula. However, it must be understood that esophageal atresia may occur as a separate malformation and that tracheoesophageal fistula without esophageal atresia also occurs. With an isolated fistula, polyhydramnios would not likely be present because amniotic fluid could pass to the stomach and intestines.

8.  D  The bronchi are derived from divisions of the lung bud, called bronchial (lung) buds. These buds differentiate into the bronchi and their ramifications in the lungs.

9.  A  Atresia or lack of continuity of the esophagus may be encountered as a separate congenital malformation. Commonly, esophageal atresia is associated with tracheoesophageal fistula. An over-all incidence of these associated malformations of one in 2200 newborn infants is generally accepted. About two-thirds of the cases occur in males. Infants present with excessive saliva, gagging, vomiting if fed, and cyanosis. Aspiration of gastric contents is responsible for the severe pulmonary symptoms.

10.  C  The variety of tracheoesophageal fistula illustrated is the most common (about 90 percent of cases). The fistula results from incomplete fusion of the tracheoesophageal folds. This canal forms at the site of the defective tracheoesophageal septum and permits communication between the esophagus and the trachea. The commonly associated esophageal atresia probably results from incomplete recanalization of the upper part of the esophagus.

11.  C  In the usual variety of tracheoesophageal fistula, associated with the inferior end of the esophageal atresia, there is a fistulous connection between the lower esophagus and the trachea (as illustrated). Not only does this fistula allow gastric contents to enter the lungs, causing severe pulmonary symptoms, but it permits air to enter the gastrointestinal tract. As a result, the abdomen rapidly becomes distended and the intestines promptly fill with air.

12.  D  An excess of amniotic fluid is commonly associated with esophageal atresia and tracheoesophageal fistula because amniotic fluid cannot pass to the intestines for absorption and subsequent transfer to the placenta for disposal. Polyhydramnios is also often associated with meroanencephaly (partial absence of the brain), possibly because the fetus lacks the neural control for swallowing amniotic fluid.

13.  E  The tracheal cartilages develop from the splanchnic mesenchyme surrounding the laryngotracheal tube. This mesenchyme also gives rise to the connective tissue and smooth muscle of the trachea.

14.  C  The type II alveolar cells, the secretory cells of the lining epithelium, produce the surface-active agent called surfactant. These cells are believed to begin producing surfactant at about 24 weeks.

15. D  A tracheoesophageal fistula (connection between the trachea and the esophagus) occurs about once in 2500 births, predominantly in males.  In 90 percent of cases this malformation is assocated with esophageal atresia.

16. C  Surfactant is a substance produced by the type II alveolar cells that is capable of lowering the surface tension at the air-alveolar surface, thereby maintaining patency of the alveoli and preventing atelectasis (imperfect expansion or collapse of the lungs).

17. A  The longitudinal laryngotracheal groove is a diverticulum of the endodermal floor of the primitive pharynx, caudal to the hypobranchial eminence (primordium of the posterior one-third of the tongue and of the epiglottis).  The endodermal lining of this groove gives rise to the epithelium and glands of the larynx, trachea and bronchi, and to the pulmonary lining epithelium.

18. C  Hyaline membrane disease, a common cause of death in the perinatal period, is associated with an absence or deficiency of surfactant (a surface-tension-lowering agent).  In this disease, which occurs particularly in babies born prematurely, a membrane-like structure lines the respiratory bronchioles, alveolar ducts and alveoli.  Because of the deficiency of surfactant, there is a tendency for the alveoli to collapse (atelectasis).

19. B  The parietal pleura develops from the mesoderm that lines the thoracic body wall.  As the lungs invaginate the pericardioperitoneal cavities (primitive pleural cavities), the space between the parietal and visceral layers of pleura is reduced to a narrow interval.

20. D  The left bronchial bud, together with the surrounding splanchnic mesenchyme, gives rise to the left lung.  At the stage shown, the bronchial buds represent the two lobes of the left lung.

21. B  The endodermal lining of the middle portion of the laryngotracheal tube gives rise to the epithelium and glands of the trachea.  The cartilage, connective tissue and smooth muscle are derived from the surrounding splanchnic mesenchyme.

22. A  The pericardioperitoneal canal connects the pericardial cavity and the peritoneal cavity during the fourth and fifth weeks.  Following division of the intraembryonic coelom into three separate cavities, these canals become the pleural cavities.

23. A  The future right pleural cavity is represented by the right pericardio-peritoneal canal.  The developing lungs grow into the splanchnic mesoderm of the medial walls of the pericardioperitoneal canals.

24. C  The splanchnic mesenchyme surrounding the developing lungs gives rise to the bronchial musculature and cartilaginous rings, and to the pulmonary connective tissue and capillaries.  The splanchnic mesenchyme also gives rise to the visceral pleura covering the lungs.

25. E  The pleural cavities are lined externally by a layer of somatic mesoderm;

subsequently this layer becomes the parietal pleura.  The invagination of the lungs into the developing pleural cavities is so complete that the space between the visceral and parietal layers of pleura becomes greatly reduced.

---

NOTES:

# THE DIGESTIVE SYSTEM

## O B J E C T I V E S

BE ABLE TO:

o     Construct and label diagrams illustrating the formation of the
      primitive gut by the incorporation of the dorsal part of the yolk
      sac into the embryo.
o     List the derivatives of the foregut.
o     Describe the rotation of the stomach and the formation of the
      omental bursa (lesser sac of the peritoneum).
o     Describe the development of the duodenum, liver, biliary
      apparatus, pancreas, and spleen.
o     List the derivatives of the midgut and illustrate herniation,
      rotation, reduction, and fixation of the midgut.
o     Write brief notes on: pyloric stenosis; omphalocele; incomplete
      rotation and volvulus of the midgut; intestinal stenosis and
      atresia; and Meckel's diverticulum.
o     List the derivatives of the hindgut.
o     Describe partitioning of the cloaca.
o     Describe development of the anal canal and write short notes on
      imperforate anus and anorectal agenesis with fistula.

## F I V E - C H O I C E   C O M P L E T I O N   Q U E S T I O N S

DIRECTIONS:  Each of the following statements or questions is followed by five
suggested responses or completions.  SELECT THE ONE BEST ANSWER in each case and
then circle the appropriate letter at the right of each question.

1. As the stomach acquires its adult shape, it rotates around
   its longitudinal axis.  Which of the following events does
   not result from this rotation?

   A.  The ventral border of the stomach moves to the right.
   B.  The dorsal border of the stomach moves to the left.
   C.  The dorsal mesogastrium is carried to the left.
   D.  The dorsal part of the stomach grows rapidly.
   E.  The duodenum slowly rotates to the right.          A B C D E

<u>SELECT THE ONE BEST ANSWER</u>

2. Derivatives of the caudal portion of the embryonic foregut are mainly supplied by which of the following arteries?

   A. Superior mesenteric
   B. Inferior mesenteric
   C. Gastroepiploic
   D. Celiac
   E. Right gastric

   A B C D E

3. Each of the following statements about the developing duodenum is true <u>except</u>:

   A. It is a derivative of the foregut and midgut.
   B. The yolk stalk is attached to the apex of the duodenal loop.
   C. It is supplied by branches of the foregut and midgut arteries.
   D. It becomes C-shaped as the stomach rotates.
   E. Its lumen is temporarily obliterated by epithelial cells.

   A B C D E

4. Hematopoiesis begins in the liver during the ____ week.

   A. third
   B. fourth
   C. fifth
   D. sixth
   E. seventh

   A B C D E

5. The most common type of anorectal malformation is

   A. anal stenosis
   B. ectopic anus
   C. anorectal agenesis
   D. anal agenesis
   E. persistent anal membrane

   A B C D E

6. The anal membrane usually ruptures at the end of the ____ week.

   A. fifth
   B. sixth
   C. seventh
   D. eighth
   E. ninth

   A B C D E

7. Pyloric stenosis is characterized by vomiting, usually starting in the second or third week after birth. The narrowing of the pyloric lumen results primarily from

   A. hypertrophy of the longitudinal muscular layer
   B. a diaphragm-like narrowing of the pyloric lumen
   C. hypertrophy of the circular muscular layer
   D. persistence of the solid stage of pyloric development
   E. a so-called 'fetal vascular accident' in the pylorus

   A B C D E

## SELECT THE ONE BEST ANSWER

8. The junction of the endodermal epithelium of the hindgut
   and the ectodermal epithelium of the proctodeum or anal
   pit is believed to be indicated by the

   A. pectinate line
   B. levator ani muscle
   C. white line
   D. external sphincter
   E. superior ends of the
      anal columns

   A B C D E

9. All the following statements about a Meckel's diverticulum
   are true except:

   A. It is a common malformation of the small intestine.
   B. It may become a leading point for an intussuception.
   C. Hemorrhage is a common sign of it during infancy.
   D. It is located on the mesenteric side of the ileum.
   E. Gastric mucosa is the most common ectopic tissue in it.

   A B C D E

10. Anorectal agenesis is more common in males than females and
    is usually associated with a rectourethral fistula. The
    embryological basis of the fistula is

    A. failure of the proctodeum to develop
    B. agenesis of the urorectal septum
    C. failure of fixation of the hindgut
    D. abnormal partitioning of the cloaca
    E. premature rupture of the anal membrane

    A B C D E

======================== ANSWERS, NOTES, AND EXPLANATIONS =========================

1. D  Growth of the stomach occurs during rotation, but it does not result from
   it. The faster growth of the original dorsal part of the stomach gives rise
   to the greater curvature of the stomach. Rotation of the stomach explains
   why the left vagus nerve supplies the anterior wall of the adult stomach, and
   why the right vagus innervates its posterior wall.

2. D  The celiac artery supplies derivatives of the caudal part of the embryonic
   foregut. It arises from the anterior aspect of the aorta just inferior to
   the aortic hiatus. It divides into the left gastric, the hepatic, and the
   splenic arteries which supply most of the foregut derivatives (inferior part
   of the esophagus, stomach, superior part of the duodenum, liver, pancreas,
   and biliary apparatus). If you chose C or E, you selected a correct answer
   because they supply some foregut derivatives. However, D is the best answer
   because it provides the main blood supply to the caudal part of the foregut.

3. B  The yolk stalk (vitelline duct) is attached to the apex of the midgut loop
   (future terminal part of ileum). The junction of the foregut and midgut
   parts of the duodenum, is located just distal to the point of entrance of the
   bile duct (common bile duct). Failure of the duodenum to recanalize results

in stenosis (narrowing) or atresia (blockage) of the duodenum. Atresia occurs about twice as often as stenosis. Infants with duodenal atresia usually vomit green fluid (because of the presence of bile). If the obstruction is superior to the point of entrance of the bile duct, however, the vomitus will not be stained with bile.

4.  D  Hematopoiesis (blood formation) begins in the mesenchyme of the yolk sac and allantois during the third week, but does not begin in the embryonic mesenchyme until the sixth week. Hemopoiesis occurs chiefly in the liver and spleen. Later, blood formation occurs in bone marrow and lymph nodes, in which sites it continues after birth.

5.  C  In most anorectal malformations, the rectum ends superior to the anal canal and levator ani muscles. Usually there is a fistulous connection with the urethra in males and the vagina in females. These defects produce intestinal obstruction because the fistulas seldom provide an adequate escape for gas and meconium (the dark green fecal material of the newborn).

6.  C  The anal membrane usually ruptures at the end of the seventh week. Imperforate anus resulting from failure of the anal membrane to perforate is uncommon. This type of imperforate anus consists of a septal occlusion of an otherwise normal anal canal. Some form of imperforate anus, usually anorectal agenesis, occurs about once in 5000 births and is much more common in males than females. The reason for this sex difference is not known.

7.  C  Pyloric stenosis is common, especially in males (about 1 in 200). The pylorus is elongated and thickened to as much as twice its usual size. Usually, forceful peristaltic waves of the gastric wall may be observed. The cause of pyloric stenosis is unknown, but hereditary factors are certainly involved. An acquired factor also appears to be involved in the pathogenesis of this 'tumor', but its nature is unknown.

8.  A  The former site of the anal membrane and thus the junction of the hindgut and the anal pit (proctodeum) is believed to be indicated by the irregular pectinate line (pectin, Latin for comb). The anal valves are attached along this line. Because of the different origins of the superior and inferior parts of the anal canal, the blood and nerve supply of the two parts differ. The inferior part of the anal canal, inferior to the pectinate line, is supplied by somatic sensory cutaneous fibers which respond immediately to painful stimuli, such as the prick of a needle. Thus, injection of a hemorrhoidal vein in the therapy of internal hemorrhoids is given superior to the pectinate line, where the mucosa is relatively insensitive to pain.

9.  D  Diverticula of the ileum, usually called Meckel's diverticula, are always on the antimesenteric border of the ileum because they represent a persistent portion of the yolk stalk (vitelline duct), which attaches to the ventral side of the midgut loop. If a Meckel's diverticulum inverts, it may serve as a leading point for an intussusception (inversion of the diverticulum and ileum into the lumen of the ileum). Bleeding of a diverticulum arises from the peptic ulcer in or adjacent to the ectopic gastric mucosa, usually at the neck of the diverticulum.

10. D  Normally the urorectal septum, a mesenchymal septum or wedge between the

allantois and the hindgut, grows caudally and fuses with the cloacal membrane. This partition divides the cloaca into the rectum dorsally and the urogenital sinus ventrally. Failure of the lateral infoldings of the cloaca, produced by caudal extensions of the urorectal septum, to fuse completely at all levels, results in communication between the rectum and the urogenital sinus. The urogenital sinus in males gives rise to the urinary bladder and almost all the urethra. Thus the fistula connects the rectum with the bladder (rectourethral fistula). In females the urogenital sinus also gives rise to the vagina; rectovaginal fistulas are most commonly associated with anorectal agenesis in females.

## MULTI-COMPLETION QUESTIONS

DIRECTIONS: In each of the following questions or incomplete statements ONE OR MORE of the completions is correct. At the lower right of each question, circle A if 1, 2, and 3 are correct; B if 1 and 3 are correct; C if 2 and 4 are correct; D if only 4 is correct; and E if all are correct.

1. Ligaments derived from the dorsal mesogastrium include:

   1. falciform
   2. gastrolienal

   3. hepatogastric
   4. phrenicolienal          A B C D E

2. Correct statements about development of the duodenum include:

   1. Most of its ventral mesentery disappears.
   2. It is derived from the foregut and midgut.
   3. Atresia is common distal to the duodenal papilla.
   4. Its lumen is obliterated by epithelial cells.          A B C D E

3. Ligaments derived from the ventral mesentery include:

   1. falciform
   2. hepatoduodenal

   3. hepatogastric
   4. coronary          A B C D E

4. Structures derived from the midgut include the:

   1. ileum
   2. vermiform appendix

   3. cecum
   4. descending colon          A B C D E

5. False statements about a Meckel's diverticulum include:

   1. may be attached to the umbilicus by a fibrous cord
   2. usually within 40 to 50 cm of the ileocecal valve
   3. hemorrhage from this diverticulum may occur
   4. usually located on the mesenteric side of the ileum          A B C D E

| A | B | C | D | E |
|---|---|---|---|---|
| 1,2,3 | 1,3 | 2,4 | only 4 | all correct |

6. Correct statements about rotation and fixation of the midgut include:

    1. The midgut loop undergoes 270 degrees of rotation.
    2. When viewed from the front, the gut rotates counter-clockwise.
    3. Most of the duodenum becomes retroperitoneal.
    4. The yolk stalk is temporarily attached to the jejunum.

    A B C D E

7. Structures communicating with the cloaca include the:

    1. hindgut
    2. mesonephric duct
    3. allantois
    4. yolk stalk

    A B C D E

8. Incomplete rotation and failure of fixation of the midgut may result in which of the following malformations?

    1. Mixed rotation
    2. Midgut volvulus
    3. Subhepatic cecum
    4. Paraduodenal hernia

    A B C D E

9. Correct statements about intestinal atresia include:

    1. Atresias are most common in the ileum.
    2. Duodenal atresia may be associated with polyhydramnios.
    3. Atresias are usually associated with vomiting.
    4. Atresia is less common than stenosis.

    A B C D E

10. Correct statements about development of the pancreas include:

    1. Most of the pancreas develops from the dorsal pancreatic bud.
    2. Part of the head of the pancreas is derived from the ventral pancreatic bud.
    3. The main pancreatic duct forms from the ducts of both pancreatic buds.
    4. The islets of Langerhans are derived from splanchnic mesenchyme.

    A B C D E

11. Biliary atresia causes jaundice and liver enlargement within a few weeks after birth. The stools are white or clay colored and the urine is dark in color. Probable causes of this congenital malformation include:

    1. failure of recanalization of the extrahepatic ducts
    2. agenesis of the cystic duct
    3. infection during the perinatal period
    4. failure of the gallbladder to form

    A B C D E

| A | B | C | D | E |
|---|---|---|---|---|
| 1,2,3 | 1,3 | 2,4 | only 4 | all correct |

12. An infant presents with a chronic discharge from the umbilicus. The embryological basis of this discharge could be an

1. umbilico-ileal fistula
2. urachal sinus
3. umbilical sinus
4. urachal fistula

A B C D E

======================= ANSWERS, NOTES, AND EXPLANATIONS =========================

1. C  **2 and 4 are correct.**  The gastrolienal (gastrosplenic) and lienorenal ligaments are derivatives of the dorsal mesogastrium; the gastrocolic and phrenicocolic ligaments have a similar origin. The falciform and hepato-gastric ligaments are derived from the ventral mesentery.

2. E  **All are correct.**  The smaller remaining part of the ventral mesentery be-comes the hepatoduodenal ligament. The free border of this ligament forms the ventral border of the epiploic foramen. The junction of the parts of the duodenum derived from the foregut and midgut is at the apex of the C-shaped embryonic duodenal loop. Because the lumen of the duodenum is normally occluded during part of the second month, failure of recanalization results in atresia (complete blockate) or stenosis (partial blockage), most often distal to the duodenal papilla.

3. E  **All are correct.**  The ventral mesentery is a thin, doubled-layered mem-brane that initially extends from the ventral wall of the primitive gut to the ventral abdominal wall. Most of it disappears soon after it forms in the fourth week, except where it is attached to the caudal part of the foregut (region of the stomach and the superior part of the duodenum). When the liver develops between its layers, the ventral mesentery between the dia-phragm and the abdominal wall becomes the falciform ligament. Between the diaphragm and the liver, the mesentery becomes the coronary and triangular ligaments.

4. A  **1, 2, and 3 are correct.**  The small intestines are derived from the midgut, except for the superior part of the duodenum (i.e., cranial to the entrance of the bile duct) which is derived from the foregut. The large intestines are also derived from the midgut, except for the left end of the transverse colon, the descending colon, the rectum, and the upper part of the anal canal; these parts are derived from the hindgut.

5. D  **4 is a false statement.**  Because of its origin from the proximal end of the yolk stalk, a Meckel's diverticulum must arise from the antimesenteric side of the ileum, a fact which distinguishes it from a duplication of the intestine. Its distal end usually lies free, but some are attached to the umbilicus by a fibrous cord. Signs and symptoms from a Meckel's diverticulum can arise at any age, but they occur most frequently during infancy.

141

6. A <u>1, 2, and 3 are correct.</u> The yolk stalk is initially attached to the apex of the midgut loop. After this portion of the midgut develops, the yolk stalk is attached to the ileum. If a portion of this stalk persists, a Meckel's diverticulum forms. It is of clinical significance because it sometimes bleeds or causes symptoms mimicking appendicitis.

7. A <u>1, 2, and 3 are correct.</u> The mesonephric ducts open into the cloaca and into the urogenital sinus after partitioning of the cloaca. In the uncommon malformation known as persistent cloaca, resulting from failure of partitioning of the cloaca, the large bowel, ureters, ejaculatory ducts (in males) and vagina (in females) open into the cloaca.

8. E <u>All are correct.</u> Incomplete rotation of the midgut, often incorrectly called malrotation, represents failure of the midgut loop to rotate completely. Incomplete rotation of the midgut is often associated with imperfect fixation of the intestines. Incomplete rotation may be responsible for partial or complete obstruction of the small intestine. Often the cecum fails to reach the right lower quadrant and the peritoneal bands fixing it to the posterior abdominal wall cross over and may partially obstruct the duodenum. Volvulus (twisting) of the intestine is present in a majority of cases of incomplete rotation because of hypermobility of the gut.

9. A <u>1, 2, and 3 are correct.</u> Atresia of the intestine is more serious and is more common than intestinal stenosis. The obstruction occurs most frequently in the ileum (about 50 percent of cases); next in the duodenum (about 25 percent of cases). In high intestinal obstruction (i.e., in the duodenum), polyhydramnios (excess of amniotic fluid) is usually present because the fetus is unable to absorb amniotic fluid that is swallowed and pass it via its blood to the placenta for excretion.

10. A <u>1, 2, and 3 are correct.</u> The islets of Langerhans develop from endodermal buds from the foregut, as do the pancreatic acini. These masses of cells develop during the 13- to 16-week period and begin to produce insulin at about 20 weeks.

11. B <u>1 and 3 are correct.</u> Initially the extrahepatic biliary apparatus is composed of solid cords; ducts form as these cords acquire lumina. If canalization fails to occur, extrahepatic biliary atresia results. It is also believed that blockage (atresia) or narrowing (stenosis) of extrahepatic bile ducts can result from liver disease during the fetal period and from perinatal hepatitis. Death will occur in all cases of biliary atresia that cannot be surgically corrected.

12. E <u>All are correct.</u> All these congenital malformations could produce a chronic drainage of fluid from the umbilicus. A urachal fistula, connected to the urinary bladder, could cause drainage of urine at the umbilicus. The umbilico-ileal fistula, if large enough, could permit drainage of fecal material from the ileum. In some cases evagination of the ileum may occur, i.e., the ileum becomes turned inside out and protrudes at the umbilicus. This is a serious complication. A vitelline cyst connected to the umbilicus by the patent distal end of the yolk stalk could discharge its secretions at the umbilicus.

# FIVE-CHOICE ASSOCIATION QUESTIONS

DIRECTIONS: Each group of questions below consists of a numbered list of descriptive words or phrases accompanied by a diagram with certain parts indicated by letters, or by a list of lettered headings. For each numbered word or phrase, SELECT THE LETTERED PART OR HEADING that matches it correctly. Then insert the letter in the space to the right of the appropriate number. Sometimes more than one numbered word or phrase may be correctly matched to the same lettered part or heading.

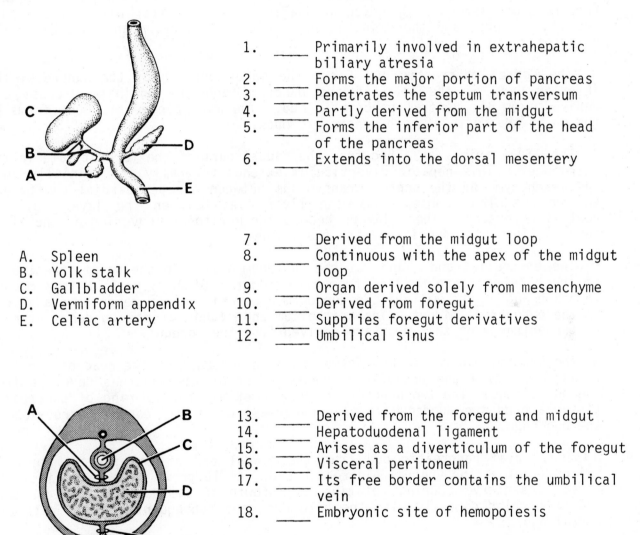

1. _____ Primarily involved in extrahepatic biliary atresia
2. _____ Forms the major portion of pancreas
3. _____ Penetrates the septum transversum
4. _____ Partly derived from the midgut
5. _____ Forms the inferior part of the head of the pancreas
6. _____ Extends into the dorsal mesentery

A. Spleen
B. Yolk stalk
C. Gallbladder
D. Vermiform appendix
E. Celiac artery

7. _____ Derived from the midgut loop
8. _____ Continuous with the apex of the midgut loop
9. _____ Organ derived solely from mesenchyme
10. _____ Derived from foregut
11. _____ Supplies foregut derivatives
12. _____ Umbilical sinus

13. _____ Derived from the foregut and midgut
14. _____ Hepatoduodenal ligament
15. _____ Arises as a diverticulum of the foregut
16. _____ Visceral peritoneum
17. _____ Its free border contains the umbilical vein
18. _____ Embryonic site of hemopoiesis

A. Pyloric stenosis
B. Anorectal agenesis
C. Esophageal atresia
D. Omphalocele
E. Polyhydramnios

19. _____ Faulty partitioning of foregut
20. _____ Herniation of intestines
21. _____ Causes projectile vomiting
22. _____ Duodenal obstruction
23. _____ Most common malformation
24. _____ Faulty partitioning of cloaca

======================= ANSWERS, NOTES, AND EXPLANATIONS =========================

1.  B  In extrahepatic biliary atresia, parts of the hepatic ducts and the bile duct are not canalized.  Portions of the bile ducts are blocked (atresia); other parts may have narrow lumina (stenosis).  These malformations are not rare, nor are they common.  The extrahepatic system of ducts develops as solid cords that normally soon become canalized.  When this fails to occur, atresia results.  If the lumen forms but is small, stenosis is present.  Congenital atresia of the bile ducts may be caused by noxious agents acting during the development of the bile duct system.  There is little evidence that this malformation is hereditary; it occurs very rarely in siblings (brothers or sisters).  Jaundice gradually increases after birth; the stools are clay colored and the urine is dark brown in color. Can you explain the basis of these observations?

2.  D  The dorsal pancreatic bud forms the major portion of the pancreas; the inferior part of the head of the pancreas and the uncinate process are derived from the ventral pancreatic bud.  The main pancreatic duct forms by fusion of the ducts of both pancreatic buds.

3.  C  The liver arises as a bud from the caudal part of the foregut late in the third week.  This hepatic diverticulum extends ventrally and cranially into the mesenchyme of the septum transversum between the pericardial cavity and the yolk stalk.  Subsequently the liver lies between the layers of the ventral mesentery.  These layers become the peritoneal covering of the liver and the ligaments associated with the liver.

4.  E  The epithelium and glands of the duodenum distal to the point of entrance of the bile duct are derived from the midgut.  Other layers of the mucous membrane and of the wall of the duodenum are derived from mesenchyme adjacent to the endodermal midgut.  The epithelium and glands of the duodenum cranial to the entrance of this duct are derived from the foregut.

5.  A  The ventral pancreatic bud forms the inferior part of the head of the pancreas, including the uncinate process.  Most of the pancreas develops from the dorsal bud.  The two pancreatic buds sometimes form a ring of pancreatic tissue around the duodenum (anular pancreas) which may cause obstruction of the duodenum.

6.  D  The dorsal pancreatic bud from the caudal end of the foregut appears, slightly before the ventral pancreatic bud.  As it grows it extends into the dorsal mesentery.  During rotation and growth of the duodenum, the ventral bud is carried dorsally with the bile duct and subsequently fuses with the dorsal bud.

7.  D  The vermiform appendix is derived from the cecal diverticulum, an outpouching from the antimesenteric side of the midgut loop.  The distal end of the cecum does not grow rapidly; thus the appendix forms.  At birth the appendix is relatively longer than in the adult, and is continuous with the apex of the cecum.

8.  B  The yolk stalk is attached to the apex of the midgut loop.  The other end

144

of this stalk is attached to the remnant of the yolk sac, located near the placenta. The yolk stalk normally degenerates at the end of the embryonic period, but in about two percent of persons the proximal part of it persists as a Meckel's diverticulum.

9.   A   The spleen is derived from a condensation of mesenchymal cells between the layers of the dorsal mesogastrium. The splenic artery is a branch of the foregut (celiac) artery; this explains why it gives off pancreatic branches, short gastric arteries, and the left gastroepiploic artery. Recall that the stomach and pancreas are foregut derivatives.

10.   C   The gallbladder is derived from the foregut. The hepatic diverticulum from the foregut divides into two parts; the larger cranial part gives rise to the liver and the caudal part gives rise to the gallbladder.

11.   E   The celiac artery carries blood from the aorta to the foregut derivatives (inferior end of the esophagus, stomach, liver, part of the duodenum, gallbladder, and part of the pancreas). The celiac artery also supplies the spleen which develops from mesenchyme in the dorsal mesentery of the stomach.

12.   B   An umbilical sinus represents a remnant of the distal portion of the yolk stalk at the umbilicus. A remnant of the proximal portion of the yolk stalk is much more common and gives rise to a Meckel's diverticulum. Umbilical sinuses are lined by intestinal mucosa and secrete a mucoid material. They may be attached to the ileum by a fibrous cord (a remnant of the proximal portion of the yolk stalk).

13.   B   The duodenum is derived from the caudal part of the foregut and the cranial part of the midgut. The junction of the foregut and midgut is at the apex of the embryonic duodenal loop, and is indicated in the adult by the point of entrance of the bile duct. Because of its dual origin, the duodenum is supplied by both the foregut (celiac) and midgut (superior mesenteric) arteries.

14.   A   The ventral mesentery between the cranial or superior part of the duodenum and the liver persists, and gives rise to the hepatoduodenal ligament. The remainder of the ventral mesentery of the foregut gives rise to the hepatogastric ligament, the peritoneal covering of the liver, the falciform ligament, and the coronary and triangular ligaments of the liver. The superior part of the duodenum is the only part of the intestines which has a ventral mesentery.

15.   D   The liver arises as a bud or diverticulum from the caudal end of the foregut. The proliferating endodermal cells give rise to interlacing cords of cells which become the liver parenchyma. The fibrous and hemopoietic tissue are derived from splanchnic mesenchyme.

16.   C   The visceral peritoneum of the liver is continuous with the hepatoduodenal ligament. This peritoneum is also continuous with the hepatogastric and falciform ligaments.

17.   E   The umbilical vein passes in the inferior free border of the falciform ligament on its way to the liver with well oxygenated blood from the placen-

ta. Within the liver the umbilical vein is broken up by the proliferating hepatic cords. The hepatic sinusoids are derived from remnants of the umbilical and vitelline veins. The adult derivative of the extrahepatic portion of the umbilical vein is the ligamentum teres (round ligament) of the liver.

18.  D  The liver is an important site of blood formation in the embryo and early fetus. Hemopoiesis begins in the liver during the sixth week; prior to this, blood formation takes place in the extraembryonic mesenchyme of the yolk sac and allantois. Blood is later formed in the spleen, bone marrow, and lymph nodes. Blood formation continues after birth in the last two sites.

19.  C  Esophageal atresia may occur as an isolated malformation, resulting from failure of canalization of the esophagus, but most often it is associated with tracheoesophageal fistula. In over 90 percent of cases of this type of fistula, the esophagus ends blindly. The fistula between the inferior end of the esophagus and the trachea results from faulty or incomplete partitioning of the foregut into the esophagus and the laryngotracheal tube. Incomplete formation of the tracheoesophageal septum at any level may give rise to a fistula.

20.  D  Omphalocele is a congenital protrusion or herniation of the intestines through a large defect in the anterior abdominal wall at the umbilicus. This malformation is believed to result from failure of the intestines to return from the umbilical cord during the tenth week. The hernial mass is covered by a thin transparent membrane, composed of peritoneum internally and amnion externally (from amniotic covering of the umbilical cord).

21.  A  Pyloric stenosis (narrowing of the distal opening of the stomach) results from hypertrophy of the muscle fibers of the pylorus, principally the circular musculature. The typical clinical picture is an infant who appears normal at birth, but within a week or more there is a gradual onset of vomiting which progresses to a projectile type.

22.  E  High intestinal obstruction (e.g., duodenal atresia) is frequently an accompaniment of polyhydramnios. Excessive amniotic fluid is also associated with meroanencephaly (partial absence of the brain) and esophageal atresia. With meroanencephaly there appears to be difficulty in swallowing. In esophageal and duodenal atresia, amniotic fluid accumulates because it is unable to pass to the intestines for absorption.

23.  A  Pyloric stenosis is the most common of all the malformations listed. It affects male infants much more often than female infants. An incidence of one in 500 births represents an approximate overall average.

24.  B  Fistulas are associated with most cases of anorectal agenesis. The fistulas are usually rectourethral in males and rectovaginal in females. Anorectal agenesis with a fistula results from faulty or incomplete partitioning of the cloaca by the urorectal septum into the rectum and urogenital sinus.

---

NOTES

# THE URINARY SYSTEM

## O B J E C T I V E S

BE ABLE TO:

---

o   Discuss the development of the three sets of excretory organs, with special emphasis on the development of the permanent kidneys.

o   Construct and label diagrams illustrating positional changes of the kidneys during development, briefly describing congenital abnormalities of position and of the renal vessels.

o   Explain, with the aid of diagrams, the formation of the urinary bladder and urethra in both sexes.

o   Describe the embryological basis of: duplications of the superior part of the urinary tract, ectopic ureteral orifices, renal ectopia, horseshoe kidneys, congenital polycystic disease of the kidney, urachal malformations, and exstrophy of the urinary bladder.

---

## F I V E - C H O I C E   C O M P L E T I O N   Q U E S T I O N S

DIRECTIONS:  Each of the following statements or questions is followed by five suggested responses or completions.  SELECT THE ONE BEST ANSWER in each case and then circle the appropriate letter at the right of each question.


1.  The human pronephros, a transitory nonfunctional 'kidney', appears early in the fourth week as a few cell clusters in the ____ region of the embryo.

    A.  occipital          D.  abdominal
    B.  cervical           E.  pelvic
    C.  thoracic                                          A B C D E

2.  The human mesonephros, a transitory functional kidney, has usually largely degenerated by the ____ week.

    A.  fifth             D.  eighth
    B.  sixth             E.  ninth
    C.  seventh                                           A B C D E

## SELECT THE ONE BEST ANSWER

3. The metanephric diverticulum appears as a dorsal outgrowth from the:

   A. mesonephric duct
   B. intermediate mesoderm
   C. urogenital sinus
   D. metanephric mesoderm
   E. cloaca                                             A B C D E

4. As the metanephric diverticulum grows dorsocranially, it becomes covered by ____ mesoderm.

   A. splanchnic           D. metanephric
   B. mesonephrogenic      E. intermediate
   C. somatic                                            A B C D E

5. Incomplete division of the metanephric diverticulum (ureteric bud) results in

   A. bifid ureter
   B. supernumerary kidney
   C. duplication of the ureter
   D. partial ureteral duplication
   E. bifid ureter and supernumerary kidney              A B C D E

6. Embryologically each uriniferous tubule consists of two parts which become confluent at the junction of the

   A. renal corpuscle and the proximal convoluted tubule
   B. proximal convoluted tubule and the loop of Henle
   C. descending and ascending limbs of the loop of Henle
   D. ascending limb of Henle's loop and the distal convoluted tubule
   E. distal convoluted tubule and the collecting tubule  A B C D E

7. Exstrophy of the bladder (ectopia vesicae) is often associated with

   A. adrenal hyperplasia
   B. urachal fistula
   C. hypospadias
   D. epispadias
   E. chromosomal abnormalities                          A B C D E

8. The metanephric diverticulum (ureteric bud) is derived from the

   A. urogenital sinus        D. somatic mesoderm
   B. splanchnic mesoderm     E. mesonephric duct
   C. metanephric mesoderm                               A B C D E

======================= ANSWERS, NOTES, AND EXPLANATIONS =========================

1. B  The rudimentary pronephric 'kidneys' appear in the cervical region. They have pronephric ducts which run caudally and open into the cloaca. The caudal parts of these ducts persist as the mesonephric ducts of the next set of kidneys which develop (the mesonephroi). In lower vertebrates, the pronephric ducts play an essential part in the induction of mesonephric tubules. They probably exert a similar influence in human embryos.

2. E  The mesonephros reaches its maximum development during the embryonic period. By the beginning of the fetal period (ninth week), most of the mesonephros has usually degenerated, except for its duct and a few tubules which persist as genital ducts in males or rudimentary structures in females. By the time the mesonephroi have degenerated, the metanephroi or permanent kidneys have formed and have begun to function.

3. A  The metanephric diverticulum (ureteric bud) develops as a dorsal outgrowth from the mesonephric duct near its entry into the cloaca. The pronephric duct, which becomes the mesonephric duct, originally developed as an outgrowth from the intermediate mesoderm.

4. D  The metanephric mass of mesoderm (metanephric blastema), derived from the nephrogenic cord, forms a mesenchymal cap over the expanded end or ampulla of the ureteric bud. This mesenchyme gives rise to the nephrons. Differentiation of the nephrons is induced by an inductor substance produced by the ampulla of the ureteric bud and later by the collecting tubules.

5. C  Incomplete division of the metanephric diverticulum (i.e., before the renal pelvis forms) usually results in the development of two ureters. One of the ureters may have an ectopic orifice, i.e., it may open into the urethra in males, or the vagina in females. Complete division of the ureteric bud (before the calyces form), results in incomplete ureteral duplication (i.e., bifid or Y-shaped ureter, or double renal pelvis).

6. E  The nephron, consisting of a renal corpuscle (glomerulus and Bowman's capsule) and its associated tubules, develops from the metanephric mass of mesoderm around the collecting tubules. The end of a distal convoluted tubule of the nephron contacts and soon becomes confluent with a collecting tubule to form a uriniferous tubule.

7. D  Exstrophy of the urinary bladder is often associated with epispadias, a condition in which the urethra opens on the dorsal surface of the penis. This severe malformation is fortunately, rare. In females with epispadias, there is a fissure in the urethra which opens on the dorsal surface of the clitoris.

8. E  The metanephric diverticulum develops as a hollow outgrowth from the mesonephric duct near its junction with the urogenital sinus. Shortly after it forms, the distal end of this outgrowth, often called the ureteric bud, expands and comes into contact with the metanephric mesoderm of the most caudal part of the nephrogenic cord.

M U L T I - C O M P L E T I O N   Q U E S T I O N S

DIRECTIONS:  In each of the following questions or incomplete statements ONE OR MORE of the completions is correct.  At the lower right of each question, circle A if 1, 2, and 3 are correct; B if 1 and 3 are correct; C if 2 and 4 are correct; D if only 4 is correct; and E if all are correct.

1.  The urinary system develops from the

    1.  intermediate mesoderm
    2.  splanchnic mesoderm
    3.  urogenital sinus
    4.  urorectal septum                        A B C D E

2.  The metanephros or permanent kidney is derived from the

    1.  paraxial mesoderm
    2.  metanephric blastema
    3.  mesonephric diverticulum
    4.  nephrogenic cord                  A B C D E

3.  Incomplete division of the ureteric bud, prior to the formation of the renal pelvis, may give rise to

    1.  ureteral duplication
    2.  a horseshoe kidney
    3.  a supernumerary kidney
    4.  crossed renal ectopia               A B C D E

4.  The epithelium of which of the following structures is derived from the endodermal urogenital sinus?

    1.  urinary bladder         3.  female urethra
    2.  ureter                4.  navicular fossa   A B C D E

5.  Exstrophy of the bladder (ectopia vesicae) is:

    1.  more common in males than in females
    2.  caused by failure of migration of mesenchymal cells
    3.  often associated with epispadias
    4.  accompanied by defective abdominal musculature   A B C D E

6.  The metanephric diverticulum

    1.  is derived from metanephric mesoderm
    2.  gives rise to the collecting system of the
       permanent kidney
    3.  gives rise to convoluted tubules and loops
       of Henle
    4.  is derived from the mesonephric duct       A B C D E

| A | B | C | D | E |
|---|---|---|---|---|
| 1,2,3 | 1,3 | 2,4 | only 4 | all correct |

7. Doubling of the collecting system of the kidney results from:

    1. incomplete division of the metanephric diverticulum
    2. a deficiency of metanephric mesoderm of blastema
    3. complete division of the metanephric diverticulum
    4. persistence of vessels that normally disappear      A B C D E

8. The excretory system of the kidney develops

    1. before the collecting system
    2. in the mesenchyme adjacent to the collecting tubules
    3. from the metanephric diverticulum or ureteric bud
    4. from the metanephric mass of mesoderm      A B C D E

9. The ureteric bud gives rise to the

    1. ureter
    2. renal pelvis
    3. collecting tubules
    4. minor and major calyces      A B C D E

======================== ANSWERS, NOTES, AND EXPLANATIONS ========================

1. A **1, 2, and 3 are correct.** The urinary system develops from the intermediate mesoderm and the cloaca. Later the cloaca is divided into the rectum dorsally and the urogenital sinus ventrally. The urogenital sinus then gives rise to the urinary bladder, urethra, and vagina in females. In males, the bladder and most of the urethra are derived from the urogenital sinus and its associated splanchnic mesenchyme.

2. C **2 and 4 are correct.** The metanephric diverticulum grows out from the dorsal wall of the mesonephric duct. The nephrogenic cord, composed of mesenchyme from the intermediate mesoderm, surrounds the dilated end of the ureteric bud and gives rise to the nephrons.

3. B **1 and 3 are correct.** Duplications of the ureter are common; supernumerary (more than two) kidneys are uncommon. These malformations result from abnormal division of the ureteric bud; incomplete division usually results in

two ureters opening from a fused kidney, but a supernumerary kidney may develop if the divided parts are widely separated. One of the ureters may have an ectopic opening, i.e., in places other than the trigone of the bladder. Complete division of the ureteric bud is likely to result in a bifid (Y-shaped) ureter, opening from separate kidneys or a fused kidney.

4.  B  1 and 3 are correct.  The epithelium of the urinary bladder and of the female urethra is derived from the urogenital sinus.  Most of the epithelium of the male urethra has a similar origin, but the epithelium of the terminal part of the penile urethra, called the navicular fossa, develops from a cord of cells which grows into the glans penis from the surface ectoderm.

5.  E  All are correct.  Exposure and protrusion of the posterior wall of the urinary bladder occurs chiefly in males.  Exstrophy of the bladder is often associated with epispadias (opening of the urethra on the dorsal surface of the penis).  Often there is also a wide separation of the pubic bones and there may be a bifid scrotum and penis.  Exstrophy results from failure of mesenchymal cells to migrate between the surface ectoderm of the anterior abdominal wall and the anterior wall of the urinary bladder during early development.  As a result, no muscle forms in this position and the thin anterior body wall and the anterior wall of the bladder rupture.  Mesenchyme later migrates into the anterior abdominal wall as far as the margin of the defect and gives rise to muscles.

6.  C  2 and 4 are correct.  The metanephric diverticulum is often called the ureteric bud to indicate that it gives rise to the urether.  This diverticulum also gives rise to the renal pelvis, the major and minor calyces, and the collecting tubules.  It has been shown experimentally that a substance released by the metanephric mesenchymal cells induces the renal pelvis to divide into the calyces, and the collecting tubules to extend from the calyces.

7.  B  1 and 3 are correct.  Incomplete division of the metanephric diverticulum results in the formation of two ureters.  Complete division of the metanephric diverticulum may also result in the formation of a supernumerary kidney if the divided portions of the diverticulum are widely separated from each other.

8.  C  2 and 4 are correct.  Contact of the ampulla or dilated end of the meta-nephric diverticulum with the metanephric mass of mesoderm appears to be essential for the development of nephrons from the mesenchyme.  The induction of nephrons is brought about by a substance released by the ampulla.  Failure of contact between the ampulla and metanephric mesenchyme results in the ureter ending blindly.

9.  E  All are correct.  The metanephric diverticula (also known as the ureteric buds) give rise to the ureters, renal pelves, calyces, and collecting tubules. They arise as outgrowths from the mesonephric ducts.

# FIVE-CHOICE ASSOCIATION QUESTIONS

DIRECTIONS: Each group of questions below consists of a numbered list of descriptive words or phrases accompanied by a diagram with certain parts indicated by letters, or by a list of lettered headings. For each numbered word or phrase, SELECT THE LETTERED PART OR HEADING that matches it correctly. Then insert the letter in the space to the right of the appropriate number. Sometimes more than one numbered word or phrase may be correctly matched to the same lettered part or heading.

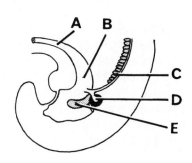

A. Renal agenesis
B. Nephrogenic cord
C. Metanephric diverticulum
D. Kidney lobes
E. Polycystic kidneys

1. ____ Urogenital sinus
2. ____ Gives rise to collecting system of the kidney
3. ____ Partitions the cloaca
4. ____ Primordium of renal pelvis and calyces
5. ____ Becomes median umbilical ligament
6. ____ Degenerates in females
7. ____ Vestigial structure in human embryos
8. ____ Embryonic kidney

9. ____ Source of nephrons
10. ____ Nonunion of nephrons and collecting tubules
11. ____ Oligohydramnios
12. ____ Mesonephric duct
13. ____ Intermediate mesoderm
14. ____ External evidence of them disappears during infancy

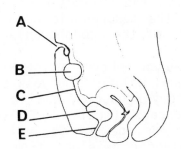

15. ____ Opens at the umbilicus
16. ____ May undergo exstrophy
17. ____ Becomes the median umbilical ligament
18. ____ Urachal sinus
19. ____ Cystic remnant of the urachus
20. ____ Short tube derived from the urogenital sinus and the adjacent splanchnic mesenchyme

======================= ANSWERS, NOTES, AND EXPLANATIONS =========================

1.  B  The urogenital sinus in the region indicated in the drawing gives rise to the epithelium of the urinary bladder.  Distally it also gives rise to the epithelium of the urethra, except for the terminal part of the spongy urethra (navicular fossa); this part is derived from the surface ectoderm.  Other parts of the walls of these structures differentiate from the adjacent splanchnic mesenchyme.

2.  D  The metanephric diverticulum gives rise to the collecting system, i.e., the ureter, renal pelvis, calcyces, and collecting tubules.  As the diverticulum grows dorsocranially, it invades the metanephric mass of mesoderm (part of the nephrogenic cord).  This mesenchyme stimulates the ureteric bud to differentiate into calyces and other parts of the collecting system of the permanent kidney.  These structures then induce the mesenchyme to differentiate into nephrons.

3.  E  The urorectal septum is a coronal sheet or wedge of mesenchyme between the allantois and the hindgut.  As it grows toward the cloacal membrane, it produces infoldings of the lateral walls of the cloaca.  When these infoldings fuse, they divide the cloaca into the rectum dorsally and the urogenital sinus ventrally.  The urorectal septum also divides the cloacal membrane into the anal membrane and the urogenital membrane.  The area of fusion of the urorectal septum with the cloacal membrane becomes the perineal body.

4.  D  The metanephric diverticulum is the primordium of the renal pelvis, the calyces, and the collecting tubules.  The metanephric mesenchyme stimulates the ampulla (future renal pelvis) of the diverticulum to divide into the calyces, and the collecting tubules to grow into the metanephric mesenchyme from the calyces.  Subsequently, these tubules contact and become confluent with the nephrons to form uriniferous tubules.

5.  A  The allantois usually becomes the urachus in the fetus and forms the median umbilical ligament in the adult.  Remnants of the allantois that do not become ligamentous may give rise to urachal sinuses, fistulas or cysts.  Urachal remnants are not detected unless they become infected.

6.  C  The mesonephros degenerates in females; almost all of it also degenerates in males.  Some caudal mesonephric tubules persist in males as the efferent ductules of the testis.  Before the mesonephros degenerates, the metanephric diverticulum grows from the mesonephric duct and forms the collecting system of the kidney.  Remnants of mesonephric tubules and the mesonephric duct may persist in females and give rise to cysts (e.g., cysts of the epoophoron).

7.  A  The allantois is a vestigial structure in the human embryo; it develops during the second week as a diverticulum from the caudal wall of the yolk sac.  In some species it serves as a reservoir for excretory products, but in the human embryo it remains small and becomes the urachus (median umbilical ligament in adults).  Although it may contribute to the apex of the urinary bladder, it is generally believed that the entire bladder develops from the urogenital sinus and the adjacent mesenchyme.

8.   C   The mesonephros is the second kidney to develop in the human embryo.  The first one (pronephros) is rudimentary, but the mesonephros is believed to function for a few weeks while the metanephros or permanent kidney is developing.

9.   B   The metanephric mesenchyme in the nephrogenic cords gives rise to nephrons.  When stimulated by a substance produced by the metanephric diverticulum, the metanephric mesenchyme begins to differentiate into nephrons.

10.  E   Congenital polycystic disease of the kidneys is transmitted on an autosomal basis.  The cysts may result from failure of the first formed rudimentary nephrons to degenerate; later these remnants may accumulate fluid and form cysts.  Cysts may also develop from detached parts of metanephric tissue which gives rise to rudimentary renal vesicles.  Cysts could also develop from nephrons which fail to establish connections with the collecting tubules.

11.  A   Oligohydramnios (an abnormally small volume of amniotic fluid) may be associated with renal agenesis (absence of kidneys).  In the newborn, renal agenesis is suggested by large low-set ears.  This type of auricle also suggests numerical chromosomal abnormalities (e.g., trisomy 18).  The fetal kidneys normally produce large amounts of urine which is excreted into the amniotic fluid.  When one or both kidneys fail to form, or there is urethral obstruction, the volume of amniotic fluid is small because urine production fails to occur or the urine cannot pass into the amniotic fluid.

12.  C   The metanephric diverticulum develops as an outgrowth of the mesonephric duct near its opening into the urogenital sinus.  This diverticulum gives rise to the ureter, renal pelvis, calyces, and collecting tubules.

13.  B   The intermediate mesoderm in the early embryo forms a longitudinal mass on each side called the nephrogenic cord.  These cords give rise to nephrons which connect with the collecting tubules formed from the ureteric buds.

14.  D   The external evidence of the kidney lobes disappears during infancy, usually by the end of the first year.  Thereafter, lobes are observed only in sections of the kidney and are defined as a medullary pyramid with its cap of cortical tissue.

15.  A   A urachal sinus may open at the umbilicus and produce a discharge.  Usually the allantois, running between the umbilicus and the urinary bladder, becomes the urachus and eventually the median umbilical ligament.  If the cranial part of the allantois remains patent, a sinus may form.  More often the caudal end of the allantois remains patent and gives rise to a sinus which may be continuous with the cavity of the urinary bladder.

16.  D   The posterior wall of the bladder may protrude through a defect in the anterior abdominal wall; this malformation is called exstrophy of the bladder.  The trigone and ureteral orifices are exposed and urine dribbles intermittently.

17.  C   The urachus, a derivative of the allantois, usually becomes a fibrous cord after birth.  Called the median umbilical ligament, it extends from the apex

of the urinary bladder to the umbilicus.

18.  A  Failure of closure of a portion of the intraembryonic part of the allantois may result in the formation of a urachal sinus that opens at the umbilicus or into the urinary bladder.  These sinuses are usually not detected unless they become infected and produce a discharge at the umbilicus or a bladder infection.

19.  B  Remnants of the urachus which do not become fibrous and form the median umbilical ligament, may accumulate fluid and become cystic.  Small cysts are commonly detected in sections of the urachus or median umbilical ligament, but cysts are usually not detected in living persons unless they become infected and enlarge.

20.  E  The urethra in the female is a short tube which extends from the urinary bladder to an external orifice.  The epithelium of the urethra is derived from the endodermal urogenital sinus; all other layers of its wall are derived from the adjacent splanchnic mesenchyme.

---

NOTES:

# THE GENITAL SYSTEM

## O B J E C T I V E S

BE ABLE TO:

_____

o    Explain sex determination in human embryos and the meaning of the
     terms chromosomal sex, genetic sex, and phenotypic sex.

o    Construct and label diagrams showing the development of: (1) the
     ovaries and testes, (2) the genital ducts, and (3) the external
     genitalia.

o    Discuss the embryological basis of hypospadias and ambiguous
     genitalia.

o    Write brief notes on: (1) the appearance, migration, and
     significance of primordial germ cells, (2) the development of
     the seminal vesicles and prostate gland, and (3) the clinically
     significant vestigial structures derived from the genital ducts.

o    Discuss the embryological basis of intersexuality and explain the
     terms true hermaphroditism and pseudohermaphroditism.

o    Describe development of the suprarenal (adrenal) glands and
     discuss congenital adrenocortical hyperplasia and its effects on
     the development of the external genitalia.

o    Construct and label diagrams showing the development of the
     inguinal canals and descent of the testes.

o    Explain the embryological basis of hydrocele and congenital
     inguinal hernia.

_____

## F I V E - C H O I C E   C O M P L E T I O N   Q U E S T I O N S

DIRECTIONS: Each of the following statements or questions is followed by five
suggested responses or completions.  SELECT THE ONE BEST ANSWER in each case and
then circle the appropriate letter at the right of each question.

1.  Primordial germ cells are first recognizable early in
    the fourth week in the

    A.  dorsal mesentery          D.  gonadal ridges
    B.  primary sex cords         E.  wall of the
    C.  wall of the yolk sac          allantois            A B C D E

## SELECT THE ONE BEST ANSWER

2. Cells of the cortical cords (secondary sex cords) derived from the coelomic ('germinal') epithelium differentiate into

   A. follicular cells
   B. stromal cells
   C. oogonia

   D. theca folliculi
   E. primordial germ
      cells            A B C D E

3. The paramesonephric ducts in female embryos gives rise to the

   A. paroophoron
   B. uterine tubes
   C. inferior part of the vagina

   D. round ligament of
      the uterus
   E. ovarian ligament   A B C D E

4. The mesonephric duct in male embryos gives rise to the

   A. duct of the epoophoron
   B. duct of Gartner
   C. ductuli efferentes

   D. ductus deferens
   E. rete testis
                    A B C D E

5. The most common cause of female pseudohermaphroditism is

   A. maternal hormone ingestion
   B. adrenocortical hyperplasia
   C. maternal arrhenoblastoma

   D. maternal progestins
   E. testicular
      feminization     A B C D E

6. Which of the following cells are derived from mesenchyme?

   A. Oogonia
   B. Interstitial cells
   C. Sertoli cells

   D. Follicular cells
   E. Spermatogonia
                    A B C D E

7. Which of the following folds give rise to labia minora?

   A. Genital
   B. Labioscrotal
   C. Urogenital

   D. Urorectal
   E. Labial
                    A B C D E

8. You are consulted about a newborn infant who was found to have chromatin positive nuclei, ambiguous external genitalia and an elevated 17-ketosteroid output. What is the most likely diagnosis?

   A. Gonadal dysgenesis with chromosomal abnormalities
   B. Female pseudohermaphroditism caused by maternal androgens
   C. Male infant with perineal hypospadias
   D. Congenital adrenocortical hyperplasia
   E. Familial male pseudohermaphroditism   A B C D E

SELECT THE ONE BEST ANSWER

9.  A newborn infant with an apparent perineal hypospadias was
    found to have chromatin negative nuclei.  Gonads were palpable
    in the inguinal canals.  The mother had previously given birth
    to an apparent female child with ambiguous external genitalia.
    This girl, now 12 years old, shows strong signs of virilization.
    What is the most likely diagnosis of the condition in the present
    infant?

    A.  Female pseudohermaphroditism      D.  Gonadal dysgenesis
    B.  Perineal hypospadias              E.  True hermaphroditism
    C.  Male pseudohermaphroditism                                A B C D E

10. The urethral groove in the female fetus usually becomes the

    A.  urethral orifice                  D.  frenulum of clitoris
    B.  urethra                           E.  vestibule of vagina
    C.  fossa navicularis                                         A B C D E

11. A 14-year-old girl was admitted because of bilateral inguinal
    masses.  She had not begun to menstruate, but showed normal
    breast development for her age.  Her external genitalia were
    feminine, the vagina was shallow, but no uterus could be pal-
    pated.  Her sex chromatin pattern was negative.  What is the
    most likely diagnosis?

    A.  Male pseudohermaphroditism        D.  Inguinal hernias
    B.  Female pseudohermaphroditism      E.  Turner syndrome
    C.  Testicular feminization                                   A B C D E


======================== ANSWERS, NOTES, AND EXPLANATIONS =========================


1.  C  The primordial germ cells are visible early in the fourth week between the
    endoderm and the mesoderm of the yolk sac, near the origin of the allantois.
    Later during the fourth week, as the yolk sac is partially incorporated into
    the embryo, the primordial germ cells migrate along the dorsal mesentery of
    the hindgut and enter the developing gonads.  They give rise to the oogonia
    and spermatogonia in the ovaries and the testes respectively.

2.  A  Cells of the coelomic ('germinal') epithelium give rise to cortical cords
    in female embryos which surround the primordial germ cells from the yolk sac.
    The primordial germ cells become oogonia and the coelomic epithelial cells
    become the follicular cells that surround the oogonia.  The coelomic
    epithelium was originally called the germinal epithelium because it was
    believed to give rise to the oogonia; however, the term germinal epithelium
    is so firmly entrenched in the literature and in people's minds that it
    probably will be called by this name for some time.

3. B  The paramesonephric ducts (formerly called mullerian ducts) give rise to the uterine tubes and uterus.  Some books state that the superior four-fifths of the vagina is also formed from the paramesonephric ducts, but it is generally believed now that the vagina is derived from the urogenital sinus and the adjacent mesenchyme.

4. D  The mesonephric ducts (formerly called wolffian ducts) give rise to the ductus epididymidis (epididymis), the ductus deferens (vas deferens), the ejaculatory duct, and the seminal vesicles.  In females the cranial end of the mesonephric duct may persist as a cystic appendix vesiculosa.  Other parts of this duct may persist as the duct of the epoophoron or as Gartner's duct, in the broad ligament along the lateral wall of the uterus and vagina.  Remnants of the duct may give rise to Gartner's duct cysts.

5. B  The congenital form of the adrenogenital syndrome results from an inborn error of metabolism.  The pituitary gland secretes excess ACTH causing hyperplasia of the fetal cortex of the suprarenal glands and an overproduction of androgens.  These hormones cause masculinization of female fetuses (female pseudohermaphroditism).  Masculinization of fetuses by hormones administered to pregnant females, or produced by maternal adrenal tumors, are uncommon causes of female pseudohermaphroditism.

6. B  The interstitial cells (of Leydig) develop from the mesenchyme located between the developing seminiferous tubules.  Some cells of this embryonic connective tissue enlarge and become grouped together to form clusters of interstitial cells.  These cells produce androgens during fetal life that masculinize the genital ducts and external genitalia of males.  The oogonia and spermatogonia develop from primordial germ cells; the follicular and Sertoli cells develop from the primary sex cords derived from the coelomic epithelium.

7. C  The urogenital folds in the female fetus usually do not fuse, but develop into the labia minora.  However, in the presence of androgenic substances they may fuse.  In males the urogenital folds fuse, closing the urethral groove and forming the spongy (penile) urethra.

8. D  An elevated 17-ketosteroid output in a chromosomal female infant with ambiguous genitalia strongly indicates congenital adrenocortical hyperplasia.  These infants have an enlarged clitoris, fused labia majora, and a persistent urogenital sinus.  The virilization results from an excessive production of androgens in the hyperplastic suprarenal (adrenal) glands.

9. C  In the case presented, the apparent female infant was a male pseudohermaphrodite.  Were it not for the family history of intersexuality, the most likely diagnosis would be hypospadias.  Inherited defects in masculinization has been reported by many investigators.  The cause of this condition is either a deficiency in the production of androgens, or a defect in end organ responsiveness to androgens.

10. E  The urogenital folds usually do not fuse in females and the urethral groove between them persists as the vestibule of the vagina (the space between the labia minora).  The urethra and vagina open into the vestibule.

11. **C** The testicular feminization syndrome is often considered a form of male pseudohermaphroditism, but these females do not have ambiguous external genitalia; hence C is the best answer. The condition is uncommon and is determined by a recessive gene. This kind of female would not pass the sex test given to females who register for the Olympics because of their chromatin negative cells. In view of her female appearance and body structure, this is unjust.

## M U L T I - C O M P L E T I O N   Q U E S T I O N S

DIRECTIONS: In each of the following questions or incomplete statements ONE OR MORE of the completions is correct. At the lower right of each question, circle A if 1, 2, and 3 are correct; B if 1 and 3 are correct; C if 2 and 4 are correct; D if only 4 is correct; and E if all are correct.

1. The epoophoron is a vestigial structure that

    1. consists of a duct and a few blind tubules
    2. corresponds to the ductus deferens
    3. lies in the broad ligament
    4. is of no clinical significance                    A B C D E

2. Congenital inguinal hernia is

    1. more common in males than females
    2. often associated with cryptorchidism
    3. a result of a persistent processus vaginalis
    4. usually of the indirect type                      A B C D E

3. The gubernaculum in the female embryo becomes the:

    1. pubocervical ligament
    2. round ligament
    3. cardinal ligament
    4. ovarian ligament                                  A B C D E

4. The labioscrotal folds in the female fetus give rise to the

    1. labia majora          3. mons pubis
    2. labial commissure      4. labia minora            A B C D E

5. Male pseudohermaphrodites usually have

    1. a 46,XY karyotype
    2. chromatin negative nuclei
    3. distinct testes
    4. male genitalia                                    A B C D E

| A | B | C | D | E |
|---|---|---|---|---|
| 1,2,3 | 1,3 | 2,4 | only 4 | all correct |

6. Hypospadias

   1. may cause ambiguous external genitalia
   2. is a relatively uncommon condition
   3. is often associated with cryptorchidism
   4. is unrelated to intersexuality          A B C D E

7. Absence of the vagina is

   1. a relatively common congenital malformation
   2. often accompanied by absence of the uterus
   3. usually associated with the Turner syndrome
   4. caused by agenesis of the sinovaginal bulbs     A B C D E

8. The processus vaginalis is

   1. a peritoneal evagination
   2. the primordium of the vagina
   3. covered by layers of the abdominal wall
   4. present only in female embryos       A B C D E

9. Correct associations concerning developing of the
   coverings of the spermatic cord include:

   1. internal oblique muscle - internal spermatic fascia
   2. internal spermatic fascia - transversalis fascia
   3. external oblique muscle - cremasteric muscle
   4. internal oblique muscle - cremasteric fascia    A B C D E

10. An infant is born with ambiguous external genitalia.
    The tentative diagnosis is female pseudohermaphroditism
    due to congenital virilizing adrenal hyperplasia.
    Which of the following observations would be consistent
    with this diagnosis?

   1. An enlarged clitoris
   2. Fused labioscrotal folds
   3. Elevated 17-ketosteroid output
   4. Chromatin positive nuclei         A B C D E

======================= ANSWERS, NOTES, AND EXPLANATIONS =========================

1. B  1 and 3 are correct. The epoophoron lies between the ovary and the
   uterine tube and corresponds to the efferent ductules and ductus epididymidis
   (epididymis) in the male. It represents persistence of a few mesonephric

tubules and part of the mesonephric duct that normally disappear in females. These remnants are clinically important because they may become distended by fluid and form parovarian cysts. The homologue of the ductus deferens is the vestigial duct of Gartner.

2. E **All are correct.** These hernias may be recognized at birth or at any age thereafter. They are located more often on the right side than the left, but frequently they are bilateral. The hernial sac (persistent processus vaginalis) is present at birth, but it often remains empty for two to three months. When the infant becomes more active, a loop of intestine may pass into the processus vaginalis, producing a bulge in the inguinal region that extends into the scrotum or towards the labium majus.

3. C **2 and 4 are correct.** In female embryos, the ligamentous gubernaculum descends from the inferior pole of the ovary, through the anterior abdominal wall (future site of inguinal canal), and attaches to the labioscrotal swelling (future labium majus). As the uterus develops, this ligament attaches to it giving rise to the ovarian ligament and the round ligament of the uterus. The round ligament passes through the inguinal canal and terminates in the labium majus.

4. A **1, 2, and 3 are correct.** The labioscrotal folds largely remain unfused to form the labia majora. They fuse posteriorly to form the posterior labial commissure and anteriorly to form the rounded elevation known as the mons pubis.

5. A **1, 2, and 3 are correct.** There is much variability of the external and internal genitalia in these males; often the external genitalia are ambiguous. Defective functioning of the testes during early fetal life is believed to cause this intersexual condition. Because of the deficiency of male hormone, persistence of parts of the paramesonephric ducts and failure of development of mesonephric ducts occur.

6. B **1 and 3 are correct.** A male infant with a severe type of hypospadias (penoscrotal or perineal) and undescended testes (cryptorchidism) cannot be distinguished easily from a virilized female infant with labioscrotal fusion and clitoral enlargement. Determination of the sex chromatin pattern and the urinary excretion of 17-ketosteroids is indicated. One of the four types of hypospadias occurs about once in 300 infants. Cryptorchidism is an associated defect in about 15 percent of cases.

7. C **2 and 4 are correct.** Absence of the vagina occurs about once in 4,000 females and is usually associated with rudimentary development or absence of the uterus. The vagina is present in females with the Turner syndrome, but the streak-like 'ovaries' are rudimentary. Absence of the vagina in otherwise normal females results from failure of the sinovaginal bulbs of the urogenital sinus to develop and form the vaginal plate.

8. B **1 and 3 are correct.** After the gubernaculum passes through the abdominal wall, an evagination of the abdominal peritoneum called the processus vaginalis projects through the abdominal wall. The processus vaginalis carries with it a covering derived from each of the layers of the abdominal wall. Before birth, the connection between the caudal end of the processus

vaginalis and the peritoneum usually becomes obliterated.

9. C  2 and 4 are correct.  As the testes and their associated structures descend, they are sheathed by fascial extensions of the layers of the abdominal wall.  The extension of the transversalis fascia becomes the internal spermatic fascia; the internal oblique muscle becomes the cremasteric fascia and muscle, and the external oblique aponeurosis forms the external spermatic fascia.

10. E  All are correct.  These findings are consistent with a diagnosis of congenital virilizing adrenal hyperplasia.  Hyperfunction of the suprarenal (adrenal) cortex resulting in excessive amounts of adrenal androgens, causes virilization of the external genitalia of female fetuses.  Of immediate concern in these infants is the possibility of adrenal crisis.  In infants with salt-losing syndromes, a weight loss (over 10 percent) occurs during the first few days.

## F I V E - C H O I C E   A S S O C I A T I O N   Q U E S T I O N S

DIRECTIONS:  Each group of questions below consists of a numbered list of descriptive words or phrases accompanied by a diagram with certain parts indicated by letters, or by a list of lettered headings.  For each numbered word or phrase, SELECT THE LETTERED PART OR HEADING that matches it correctly.  Then insert the letter in the space to the right of the appropriate number.  Sometimes more than one numbered word or phrase may be correctly matched to the same lettered part or heading.

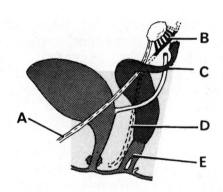

1. _____ Derivative of paramesonephric duct
2. _____ Corresponds to the epididymis
3. _____ Passes through the inguinal canal
4. _____ Composed of endodermal cells
5. _____ Derivative of the gubernaculum
6. _____ Derivative of urogenital sinus
7. _____ Epoophoron
8. _____ Gartner's duct cyst

A. Adrenal hyperplasia
B. Penile hypospadias
C. Zona reticularis
D. Neuroectoderm
E. Coelomic epithelium

9. _____ Suprarenal medulla
10. _____ Gives rise to the suprarenal cortex
11. _____ Differentiates after birth
12. _____ Unfused urogenital folds
13. _____ Ambiguous external genitalia
14. _____ Associated with chordee

## ASSOCIATION QUESTIONS

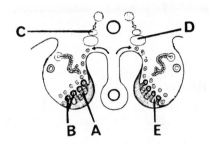

A. Urogenital folds
B. Rete testis
C. Glandular plate
D. Genital tubercle
E. External oblique aponeurosis

15. _____ Primordium of suprarenal medulla
16. _____ Gives rise to interstitial cells
17. _____ Primary sex cord
18. _____ Primordium of suprarenal cortex
19. _____ Give rise to oogonia
20. _____ Degenerates in females

21. _____ External spermatic fascia
22. _____ Gives rise to the clitoris
23. _____ Primary sex cords in males
24. _____ Hypospadias
25. _____ Navicular fossa
26. _____ Labia minora

======================= ANSWERS, NOTES, AND EXPLANATIONS =======================

1.  C  The uterine tube is a derivative of the paramesonephric duct.  The fused portions of these ducts give rise to the uterus.

2.  B  The epoophoron appears in the broad ligament between the ovary and the uterine tube.  It is a remnant of the mesonephric duct and some mesonephric tubules and is homologous with the epididymis in males.  It may become cystic and give rise to a large parovarian cyst.

3.  A  The round ligament of the uterus passes through the inguinal canal and inserts in the labium majus.  It is continuous with the ovarian ligament because they are both derived from the embryonic gubernaculum.

4.  E  The vaginal plate is composed of endodermal cells derived from the urogenital sinus.  Later the central cells of this plate break down, forming the lumen of the vagina.  Failure of this canalization to occur results in vaginal atresia.

5.  A  The round ligament is a derivative of the gubernaculum, a fibromuscular cord that passes from the inferior pole of the gonad.  It descends obliquely through the developing abdominal wall (future site of the inguinal canal), and attaches to the labioscrotal fold (future labium majus).

6.  E  The vaginal plate is derived from a pair of sinovaginal bulbs which grow out from the urogenital sinus and fuse to form a solid cord of endodermal

165

cells, called the vaginal plate. The central cells of this plate subsequently degenerate, forming the lumen of the vagina.

7.  B  The epoophoron is a vestigial structure that lies in the broad ligament between the ovary and the uterine tube. It consists of a few blind tubules connected to a short duct. If the epoophoron becomes distended with fluid, it forms a parovarian cyst. Often these are small, but some enlarge to an enormous size.

8.  D  Gartner's duct cysts are derived from remnants of caudal parts of the mesonephric duct in females. They are located between the layers of the broad ligament along the lateral wall of the uterus, or in the wall of the vagina. Gartner's duct cysts are rarely detected unless they become infected and enlarged.

9.  D  The medulla of the suprarenal gland is derived from neuroectoderm. Neural crest cells, comparable to those that form sympathetic ganglia, invade the mesodermal suprarenal cortex on its medial side and soon become surrounded by it.

10.  E  The fetal suprarenal (adrenal) cortex is derived from mesenchymal cells that arise from the coelomic epithelium. These large cells make up most of the suprarenal cortex before birth forming the massive fetal cortex. The fetal cortex gradually involutes after birth and is usually not recognizable after the first year.

11.  C  At birth the suprarenal gland consists mainly (about 80 percent) of fetal cortex. The zona reticularis of the adrenal cortex forms after birth. It is usually recognizable by the end of the third year. The other two layers of the permanent cortex (zona glomerulosa and zona fasciculata) are present at birth, but are not fully differentiated.

12.  B  Failure of the urogenital folds to fuse in males results in hypospadias. In most cases (about 80 percent), the urethra opens on the ventral surface near the junction of the glans and the body (shaft) of the penis.

13.  A  Ambiguous external genitalia often indicate virilization of a female, resulting from congenital virilizing adrenal hyperplasia. Excessive production of adrenal androgens by the hyperplastic fetal cortex of the suprarenal gland causes masculinization of the external genitalia. Generally a newborn with ambiguous genitalia, a palpable uterus, but no palpable gonads is a female pseudohermaphrodite caused by adrenocortical hyperplasia.

14.  B  Chordee, a curving downward of the penis, is often associated with hypospadias, especially with the more severe types (e.g., penoscrotal hypospadias).

15.  C  The medulla of the suprarenal gland is derived from neuroectoderm. Neural crest cells, comparable to those that give rise to sympathetic nerve cells, migrate to the developing suprarenal glands. These cells are soon encapsulated by the mesodermal suprarenal cortex and later give rise to the suprarenal medulla.

16.  E  The mesenchyme, separating the primary sex cords, gives rise to the interstitial cells. Some cells of the mesenchyme (embryonic connective tissue) enlarge and become grouped together. They produce androgens during the fetal period which stimulate development of the mesonephric ducts and inhibit development of the paramesonephric ducts. These sex hormones also cause masculinization of the external genitalia.

17.  A  The primary sex cords give rise to the seminiferous tubules, the tubuli recti, and the rete testis. They lose their connections with the surface epithelium as the tunica albuginea forms.

18.  D  The suprarenal cortex, derived from mesoderm, is first recognizable as a mass of mesenchymal cells on each side between the root of the mesentery and the developing gonad. Before birth, most of the suprarenal cortex (about 80 percent) consists of fetal cortex. This zone rapidly involutes after birth, losing about half its mass in two weeks.

19.  B  The primordial germ cells are the precursors of the oogonia in female embryos, and of spermatogonia in male embryos. The primordial germ cells come from the yolk sac to the gonads and soon become incorporated into the primary sex cords.

20.  A  The primary sex cords normally degenerate in female embryos, but during the fetal period secondary sex cords (often called cortical cords) extend from the surface epithelium into the underlying mesenchyme. Primordial germ cells are incorporated into the cortical cords and give rise to the oogonia. The follicular cells surrounding the oogonia are derived from the cortical cords.

21.  E  The external spermatic fascia is an extension of the external oblique aponeurosis. As the testis and its associated structures descend, they become ensheathed by fascial extensions of the abdominal wall. These extensions are produced by the processus vaginalis as it projects through the abdominal wall along the path formed by the gubernaculum.

22.  D  The genital tubercle elongates in both sexes to form a phallus. In females, growth of the phallus normally slows after the eighth week; it becomes the relative small clitoris. In the presence of androgenic substances (e.g., administered to the mother or produced by hyperplastic fetal suprarenal glands), however, the clitoris elongates to form a penis-like structure, and the labia majora fuse.

23.  B  The primary sex cords in male embryos condense and extend into the medulla of the developing testis. Here they branch and their ends anastomose to form the rete testis.

24.  A  Hypospadias is a common abnormal condition of the urethra (about one in 300 males) resulting from failure of fusion of the urogenital folds. In some cases the labioscrotal folds also fail to fuse and result in severe forms of hypospadias (e.g., penoscrotal and perineal hypospadias). This arrest of development is the result of an inadequate production of androgens by the fetal testes.

25.  C  The terminal portion of the penile urethra, the navicular fossa, is derived from the glandular plate. This plate is formed by an ectodermal ingrowth into the glans penis from the surface epithelium. Subsequent splitting of this plate forms a groove on the ventral surface of the glans. Closure of the urethral groove moves the external urethral orifice to the tip of the glans penis and joins this part of the spongy urethra with that formed by fusion of the urogenital folds.

26.  A  The labia minora develop from the urogenital folds. In male embryos that receive adequate amounts of androgenic hormones, the urogenital folds fuse to form the spongy urethra.

<u>NOTES</u>:

# THE CARDIOVASCULAR SYSTEM

## O B J E C T I V E S

BE ABLE TO:

---

o   Illustrate with simple labelled sketches, the events occurring between the third and sixth weeks which change the primitive heart tube into the shape that characterizes the adult heart.

o   Explain partitioning of the primitive atrium and ventricle, discussing clinically significant atrial and ventricular septal defects.

o   Construct and label diagrams illustrating the course of the fetal circulation and the changes that normally occur at birth.

o   Summarize the major events in the transformation of the embryonic aortic arch system into the adult arterial pattern.

o   Discuss the relatively common aortic arch anomalies (especially patent ductus arteriosus and coarctation of the aorta).

o   Outline the embryological basis of the following congenital malformations: double aortic arch, right aortic arch, and retroesophageal subclavian artery.

---

## F I V E - C H O I C E   C O M P L E T I O N   Q U E S T I O N S

DIRECTIONS: Each of the following statements or questions is followed by five suggested responses or completions.  SELECT THE ONE BEST ANSWER in each case and then circle the appropriate letter at the right of each question.

1.   Incomplete fusion of the endocardial cushions is usually associated with which of the following types of atrial septal defect (ASD)?

   A.  secundum type ASD
   B.  primum type ASD
   C.  common atrium
   D.  probe patent ASD
   E.  sinus venosus type ASD                          A B C D E

SELECT THE ONE BEST ANSWER

2. The fetal left atrium is mainly derived from the:

   A. primitive pulmonary vein
   B. right pulmonary vein
   C. primitive atrium
   D. sinus venarum
   E. sinus venosus                           A B C D E

3. Congenital heart disease is the most common cardiac condition in childhood and most frequently results from

   A. maternal medications
   B. mutant genes
   C. rubella virus
   D. fetal distress
   E. genetic and environmental factors        A B C D E

4. The most common type of defect of the cardiac septa is

   A. secundum type ASD
   B. muscular type VSD
   C. primum type ASD
   D. membranous type VSD
   E. sinus venosus type ASD                    A B C D E

5. Closure of the foramen primum results from fusion of the

   A. septum primum and the septum secundum
   B. septum secundum and the septum spurium
   C. septum primum and the endocardial cushions
   D. septum secundum and the endocardial cushions
   E. septum primum and the right sinoatrial valve   A B C D E

6. The fetal right atrium is mainly derived from the

   A. primitive pulmonary vein
   B. right pulmonary vein
   C. primitive atrium
   D. sinus venarum
   E. sinus venosus                            A B C D E

7. The most common congenital malformation of the heart and
   great vessels associated with the congenital rubella
   syndrome is

   A. coarctation of the aorta
   B. tetralogy of Fallot
   C. patent ductus arteriosus
   D. atrial septal defect
   E. ventricular septal defect                 A B C D E

8. The cardiovascular system reaches a functional state at the end
   of the _____ week.

   A. second
   B. third
   C. fourth

   D. fifth
   E. sixth

   A B C D E

======================= ANSWERS, NOTES, AND EXPLANATIONS =======================

1. B  The primum type ASD associated with an endocardial cushion defect is the second most common type of clinically significant ASD. The incomplete form of endocardial cushion defect is relatively common, in which the septum primum does not fuse with the endocardial cushions. As a result, there is a patent foramen primum and often there is also a cleft in the anterior (or septal) leaflet of the mitral valve.

2. A  Most of the wall of the left atrium is smooth and is derived by absorption of the primitive pulmonary vein. At first a common pulmonary vein opens into the primitive left atrium, but as the atrium expands portions of this vein are incorporated into the wall of the atrium. The primitive atrium forms only a relatively small part of the adult left atrium, i.e., the left auricle.

3. E  Congenital heart disease is not usually caused by a single etiological factor. Heart malformations are found in single gene disorders, but most fit the criteria for multifactorial inheritance. Rubella virus is an agent known to be associated with patent ductus arteriosus and pulmonary stenosis. Maternal medications (e.g., thalidomide) are occasionally associated with congenital heart disease; however, most heart defects result from unknown causes, probably a complex interaction of genetic and environmental factors.

4. D  Membranous type VSD (ventricular septal defect) is the most common type of cardiac defect. Usually this defect results from failure of the membranous portion of the interventricular septum to form at the end of the seventh week.

5. C  As the septum primum grows towards the fusing endocardial cushions, the foramen primum becomes progressively smaller. Eventually the septum primum fuses with the left side of the fused endocardial cushions and obliterates the foramen primum.

6. E  Most of the wall of the right atrium is smooth and is derived by absorption of the right horn of the sinus venosus. Initially the sinus venosus opens into the right atrium but as the atrium expands, the right horn of the sinus venosus is gradually incorporated into the right atrium and becomes the smooth-walled part, called the sinus venarum. The primitive atrium is represented by the right auricle, a small muscular pouch. The smooth part (sinus venarum) and the rough part (auricle) are demarcated internally by a vertical ridge, the crista terminalis, and externally by a shallow inconspicuous groove, the sulcus terminalis.

171

7.  C  The most frequent abnormalities in the congenital rubella syndrome are congenital heart disease (especially patent ductus arteriosus and pulmonary stenosis), deafness, and blindness (cataract). These malformations result from maternal infection during the first trimester of pregnancy. Rubella infection during the second trimester can cause deafness, microcephaly and mental retardation. The influence of teratogens such as rubella on development of the heart and great vessels is well known, but the role of other viral infections and drugs is inconclusive.

8.  B  Cardiovascular development is first evident in the cardiogenic area at about 18 days. By the end of the third week, embryonic and extraembryonic vessels are connected to the heart and a slow circulation of blood has begun. When the heart begins to beat about a day later, the circulation becomes an ebb and flow type.


# M U L T I - C O M P L E T I O N   Q U E S T I O N S

DIRECTIONS:  In each of the following questions or incomplete statements ONE OR MORE of the completions is correct. At the lower right of each question, circle A if 1, 2, and 3 are correct; B if 1 and 3 are correct; C if 2 and 4 are correct; D if only 4 is correct; and E if all are correct.


1.  The fetal left atrium receives blood from the

    1.  common cardinal vein
    2.  right atrium
    3.  sinus venosus
    4.  pulmonary veins                               A  B  C  D  E

2.  The truncus arteriosus of the primitive heart

    1.  is partitioned by the aorticopulmonary septum
    2.  may persist after birth in some infants
    3.  gives rise to the aorta and the pulmonary trunk
    4.  forms part of the adult descending aorta        A  B  C  D  E

3.  The U-shaped bulboventricular loop of the primitive heart forms as a result of the

    1.  growth of the bulbus cordis and ventricle
    2.  transverse folding of the embryo
    3.  fixation of the ends of the heart
    4.  heart sinking into the pericardial cavity       A  B  C  D  E

| A | B | C | D | E |
|---|---|---|---|---|
| 1,2,3 | 1,3 | 2,4 | only 4 | all correct |

4. The bulbus cordis of the embryonic heart is represented in the adult heart by the

    1. left auricle
    2. conus arteriosus
    3. aortic sac
    4. aortic vestibule                                      A B C D E

5. The third pair of aortic arches (arteries) give rise to which of the following arteries?

    1. common carotid
    2. external carotid
    3. internal carotid
    4. subclavian                                            A B C D E

6. The sixth pair of aortic arches (arteries) develop in which of the following ways?

    1. The proximal parts form parts of the pulmonary arteries.
    2. They contribute to distal parts of the subclavian arteries.
    3. On the left the distal part persists as the ductus arteriosus.
    4. They form a large part of the arch of the aorta.     A B C D E

7. The course of the adult recurrent laryngeal nerves differs on the two sides because of differences in the transformation of the sixth aortic arch arteries. As a result the

    1. left recurrent laryngeal nerve hooks around the ligamentum arteriosum
    2. right recurrent laryngeal nerve hooks around the right subclavian artery
    3. left recurrent laryngeal nerve hooks around the arch of the aorta
    4. right recurrent laryngeal nerve hooks around the right common carotid artery                          A B C D E

8. Defects forming part of the tetralogy of Fallot include:

    1. pulmonary stenosis
    2. atrial septal defect
    3. ventricular septal defect
    4. hypertrophy of the left ventricle                    A B C D E

173

| A | B | C | D | E |
|---|---|---|---|---|
| 1,2,3 | 1,3 | 2,4 | only 4 | all correct |

9.  Events usually occurring when circulation of blood
    through the placenta ceases and the lungs begin to
    function at birth include:

    1.  blood pressure in the inferior vena cava falls
    2.  pulmonary vascular resistance falls
    3.  blood pressure in the left atrium rises
    4.  the foramen ovale closes                              A B C D E

10. Some malformations of the heart and great vessels occur much
    more frequently than others.  Which of the following malfor-
    mations are relatively common?

    1.  Ventricular septal defect
    2.  Patent ductus arteriosus
    3.  Tetralogy of Fallot
    4.  Transposition of the great arteries                   A B C D E

11. Closure of the interventricular foramen occurs around the end
    of the seventh week mainly as a result of the fusion of sub-
    endocardial tissue from which of the following sources?

    1.  endocardial cushions       3.  bulbar ridges
    2.  interventricular septum     4.  septum secundum        A B C D E

12. Patent ductus arteriosus is

    1.  a common malformation
    2.  associated with rubella infection
    3.  more frequent in females
    4.  an aortic arch malformation                           A B C D E


======================== ANSWERS, NOTES, AND EXPLANATIONS ========================


1.  C  2 and 4 are correct.  Blood from the inferior vena cava and the right
    atrium is largely directed by the lower border of the septum secundum, called
    the crista dividens, through the foramen ovale into the left atrium.  Very
    little blood enters the left atrium from the pulmonary veins because little
    blood passes to the lungs as they are not functioning.  Pulmonary vasculature
    resistance is high, thus relatively little blood from the pulmonary trunk
    enters the lungs; most of it is directed to the descending thoracic aorta by
    way of the ductus arteriosus.

2.  A  1, 2, and 3 are correct.  The aorticopulmonary septum forms during the

fifth week and divides the bulbus cordis and the truncus arteriosus into the aorta and pulmonary trunk. In about one in 150,000 infants, this septum fails to form and a single arterial vessel arises from the heart (persistent truncus arteriosus). The descending aorta is derived from the fused embryonic dorsal aortae.

3. B **1 and 3 are correct**. The arterial and venous ends of the heart are fixed by the branchial arches and the septum transversum, respectively. Because of rapid growth of the bulbus cordis and ventricle, compared to the growth of other cardiac regions, the primitive heart bends on itself forming a U-shaped loop.

4. C **2 and 4 are correct**. As the heart develops, the bulbus cordis is gradually incorporated into the walls of the ventricles. In the right ventricle it is represented by the conus arteriosus or infundibulum; in the left ventricle it becomes the aortic vestibule. Failure of the bulbus cordis to expand normally results in infundibular stenosis, or narrowing of the right ventricular outflow.

5. B **1 and 3 are correct**. The proximal parts of the third pair of aortic arch arteries give rise to the common carotid arteries; the distal portions join the dorsal aortae to form the internal carotid arteries. The external carotid arteries may form partly from the first pair of aortic arch arteries, but their origin is controversial. They probably develop independently of the aortic arch arteries.

6. B **1 and 3 are correct**. The distal parts of the pulmonary arteries are derived from buds of the sixth aortic arch arteries which grow into the developing lungs. The distal portion of the right sixth aortic arch degenerates; the distal part of the left sixth arch forms the ductus arteriosus. At birth, the ductus arteriosus narrows as a result of contraction of its muscular coat. Anatomical closure (obliteration of its lumen) of the ductus arteriosus occurs during infancy.

7. A **1, 2, and 3 are correct**. On the right, because the distal part of the right sixth aortic arch artery and the fifth aortic arch degenerate, the right recurrent laryngeal nerve moves superiorly and hooks around the proximal part of the right subclavian artery. In the fetus, the left recurrent laryngeal nerve hooks around the ductus arteriosus and the arch of the aorta. Usually the ductus arteriosus becomes the ligamentum arteriosum during infancy.

8. B **1 and 3 are correct**. Classically the four defects of the heart and great vessels are: (1) stenosis of the pulmonary tract at one or more levels; (2) a ventricular septal defect; (3) right ventricular hypertrophy; and (4) an aorta which straddles or overrides the defect at its origin. Fallot's name has been firmly established with this group of defects since 1888, when he wrote several papers showing how these defects differed from other causes of 'blue babies' (infants with cyanosis, a bluish discoloration). Tetralogy of Fallot accounts for about 10 percent of all congenital heart disease.

9. E **All are correct**. When the placental circulation ceases, the amount of blood entering the inferior vena cava and the right atrium decreases, result-

ing in a fall of blood pressure in these structures. When breathing occurs the lungs expand, the pulmonary vascular resistance falls, and more blood flows to the lungs. As a result, more blood leaves the lungs and enters the left atrium, thereby raising its pressure and closing the foramen ovale.

10. E  <u>All are correct.</u>  These are the common malformations of the heart and great vessels, listed in their usual order of frequency. These defects account for over 50 percent of the cases of congenital heart disease. Of the four conditions, tetralogy of Fallot and transposition of the great vessels are amongst the leading causes of death during infancy.

11. B  <u>1 and 3 are correct.</u>  The interventricular foramen closes as a result of proliferation of tissue from three sources: the right and left bulbar ridges and the fused endocardial cushions. These tissues grow and fuse with the superior edge of the crescentic muscular interventricular septum. While this septum may contribute to closure of the foramen, it is not considered a major source of tissue.

12. E  <u>All are correct.</u>  Patent ductus arteriosus (PDA) is one of the most common malformations of the heart and great vessels, ranking second to ventricular septal defect (VSD).

## F I V E - C H O I C E   A S S O C I A T I O N   Q U E S T I O N S

DIRECTIONS:  Each group of questions below consists of a numbered list of descriptive words or phrases accompanied by a diagram with certain parts indicated by letters, or by a list of lettered headings. For each numbered word or phrase, SELECT THE LETTERED PART OR HEADING that matches it correctly. Then insert the letter in the space to the right of the appropriate number. Sometimes more than one numbered word or phrase may be correctly matched to the same lettered part or heading.

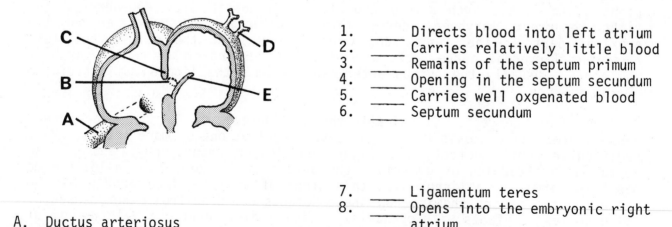

1. ____ Directs blood into left atrium
2. ____ Carries relatively little blood
3. ____ Remains of the septum primum
4. ____ Opening in the septum secundum
5. ____ Carries well oxgenated blood
6. ____ Septum secundum

7. ____ Ligamentum teres
8. ____ Opens into the embryonic right atrium
9. ____ An arterial shunt
10. ____ Floor of the fossa ovalis
11. ____ Ductus venosus
12. ____ Right recurrent laryngeal nerve

A. Ductus arteriosus
B. Septum primum
C. Right sixth aortic arch
D. Sinus venosus
E. Umbilical vein

## ASSOCIATION QUESTIONS

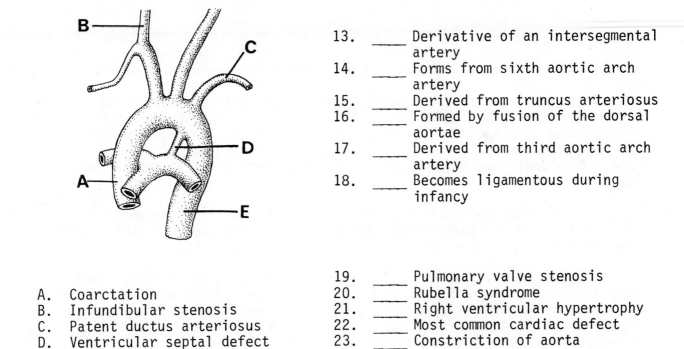

13. ____ Derivative of an intersegmental artery
14. ____ Forms from sixth aortic arch artery
15. ____ Derived from truncus arteriosus
16. ____ Formed by fusion of the dorsal aortae
17. ____ Derived from third aortic arch artery
18. ____ Becomes ligamentous during infancy

A. Coarctation
B. Infundibular stenosis
C. Patent ductus arteriosus
D. Ventricular septal defect
E. Tetralogy of Fallot

19. ____ Pulmonary valve stenosis
20. ____ Rubella syndrome
21. ____ Right ventricular hypertrophy
22. ____ Most common cardiac defect
23. ____ Constriction of aorta
24. ____ Overriding aorta

======================= ANSWERS, NOTES, AND EXPLANATIONS =========================

1. C  Blood from the inferior vena cava is directed by the inferior border of the septum secundum (crista dividens) through the foramen ovale into the left atrium.

2. D  The pulmonary veins carry relatively little blood to the left atrium before birth because the lungs are not functioning. When the lungs expand at birth and the pulmonary vascular resistance falls, there is a marked increase in pulmonary blood flow with a consequent increased flow to the left atrium through the pulmonary veins.

3. E  The remains of the septum primum are represented here by the valve of the foramen ovale. This valve is forced open by blood from the inferior vena cava which is directed through the foramen ovale by the crista dividens (inferior edge of septum secundum). The foramen ovale normally closes at birth when pressure in the left atrium rises above that in the right atrium.

4. B  The foramen ovale is a normal opening in the septum secundum. It permits well-oxygenated blood from the placenta entering via the inferior vena cava to enter the left atrium. If this opening fails to close at birth, a cardiac

malformation known as secundum type ASD exists. This is a common congenital heart defect, accounting for about eight percent of cases of congenital heart disease.

5.  A  The inferior vena cava carries well oxygenated blood from the placenta. This fetal blood returns from the placenta in the umbilical vein. About half of the blood passes through the hepatic sinusoids before entering the inferior vena cava. The other half is shunted via the ductus venosus directly from the umbilical vein to the inferior vena cava.

6.  C  The septum secundum is the second part of the interatrial septum to form. The crista dividens, its inferior border, is indicated by the pointer. It directs most of the blood from the inferior vena cava through the opening in the septum secundum (foramen ovale) into the left atrium. The smaller portion of blood, turned back by the septum secundum, enters the right ventricle.

7.  E  The intra-abdominal portion of the fetal umbilical vein becomes the adult ligamentum teres and passes from the umbilicus to the porta hepatis, where it attaches to the left branch of the portal vein.

8.  D  The sinus venosus is initially a separate chamber of the heart that opens into the caudal wall of the right atrium. The right horn of the sinus venosus becomes incorporated into the wall of the right atrium and forms the smooth-walled portion called the sinus venarum. The left horn of the sinus venosus becomes the coronary sinus.

9.  A  The ductus arteriosus is an arterial shunt that carries blood from the left pulmonary artery to the arch of the aorta before birth. Because the lungs are not functioning, most of the blood in the pulmonary artery bypasses the lungs and enters the descending aorta.

10.  B  The floor of the fossa ovalis in the interatrial septum is formed by tissue derived from the septum primum (valve of the foramen ovale). When the pressure in the left atrium rises at birth, the valve of the foramen ovale closes and later fuses with the septum secundum. It is this valvular tissue that forms the floor of the fossa ovalis.

11.  E  About half the blood coming from the placenta in the umbilical vein is shunted through the liver through the ductus venosus into the inferior vena cava. The remainder of the blood enters the liver and is carried to the inferior vena cava by the hepatic veins.

12.  C  The recurrent laryngeal nerves hook around the sixth pair of aortic arch arteries. On the right, the distal part of the sixth arch artery and the fifth aortic arch artery degenerate, leaving the right recurrent laryngeal nerve hooked around the right subclavian artery. On the left, the recurrent laryngeal nerve hooks around the ductus arteriosus (ligamentum arteriosum in the adult) and the arch of the aorta.

13.  C  The left subclavian artery, unlike the right subclavian artery, is not derived from an aortic arch artery or from the dorsal aorta. It develops

from the seventh intersegmental artery that arises from the descending aorta and moves cranially as the arch of the aorta forms.

14. D  The ductus arteriosus develops from the distal portion of the left sixth aortic arch artery.  It passes from the left pulmonary artery to the aorta and before birth carries most of the blood from the pulmonary trunk into the aorta.  The lungs are not functioning and so require little blood.  The ductus arteriosus usually constricts slightly after birth and closes anatomically during the first three months.

15. A  The proximal part of the ascending aorta is derived from the truncus arteriosus when it is divided by the aorticopulmonary septum.  The remainder of the ascending aorta develops from the aortic sac.

16. E  The descending aorta forms when the paired dorsal aortae of the embryo fuse just caudal to the heart.  The cranial portion of the right dorsal aorta normally involutes, but if it persists, a double aortic arch forms which may compress the trachea and esophagus.

17. B  The right common carotid artery is derived from the proximal part of the right third aortic arch artery.  This artery also gives rise to the internal carotid artery on this side.

18. D  The ductus arteriosus constricts slightly at birth, but is usually patent for a week or so.  Proliferation of endothelial and fibrous tissues of the ductus arteriosus usually results in its anatomical closure by the end of the third month.

19. E  Stenosis of the pulmonary tract is one of the four malformations of the heart and great vessels included in the tetralogy of Fallot.  Tetralogy of Fallot is generally regarded as the most important of the cardiac malformations that produce cyanosis.

20. C  Patent ductus arteriosus is the most common congenital malformation of the heart and great vessels associated with maternal rubella infection during the first trimester.

21. B  Enlargement and hypertrophy of the right ventricle results from high blood pressure, often resulting from pulmonary stenosis.  The narrowing may occur at the infundibulum of the right ventricle, the pulmonary valve, or less commonly in the pulmonary trunk.  E is also correct, but B is the better answer.

22. D  Ventricular septal defect (VSD) is the most common heart defect, accounting for about 22 percent of cases of congenital heart disease.  VSD may occur with quite a variety of other cardiac defects, e.g., in tetralogy of Fallot. VSD most commonly consists of an opening (1 to 15 mm in diameter) in the membranous portion of the interventricular septum.

23. A  In preductal coarctation, there is a constriction of the aorta superior to the ductus arteriosus which is usually patent.  More often, the constriction is inferior to the ductus (postductal coarctation).

24.  E  Overriding aorta or an aorta arising directly over a ventricular septal defect, and thus overriding both ventricular cavities, is an essential feature of the tetralogy of Fallot.  Persons with this group of cardiac abnormalities are cyanotic because not enough blood flows to the lungs for oxygenation.  As long as the ductus arteriosus remains patent, there is compensatory flow through it from the aorta to the pulmonary arteries.  If the ductus closes, as commonly occurs, the deficit in pulmonary circulation is increased.

---

NOTES:

# THE SKELETAL AND MUSCULAR SYSTEMS

## O B J E C T I V E S

BE ABLE TO:

o   Construct and label diagrams showing the development and early
    differentiation of a somite.
o   Discuss briefly the histogenesis of skeletal, cardiac, and smooth
    muscle.
o   Describe endochondral and intramembranous bone formation.
o   Construct and label diagrams illustrating the development of the
    different types of joint.
o   Describe the development of a typical vertebra.
o   Make and label simple sketches of the fetal skull illustrating
    the bones, fontanelles, and sutures.
o   Discuss briefly:  achondroplasia, spina bifida occulta, cervical
    and lumbar ribs, acrania, and craniosynostosis.

## F I V E - C H O I C E   C O M P L E T I O N   Q U E S T I O N S

DIRECTIONS:  Each of the following statements or questions is followed by five
suggested responses or completions.  SELECT THE ONE BEST ANSWER in each case and
then circle the appropriate letter at the right of each question.

1.  Which of the following bones is <u>not</u> mainly formed by
    endochondral ossification?

    A.  Humerus              D.  Occipital
    B.  Mandible             E.  Tibia
    C.  Hyoid                                        A B C D E

2.  Which of the following bones is completely formed by
    intramembranous ossification?

    A.  Stapes               D.  Radius
    B.  Parietal             E.  Sphenoid
    C.  Clavicle                                     A B C D E

SELECT THE ONE BEST ANSWER

3.  The most common type of accessory rib is a _____ rib.

    A.  lumbar                D.  thoracic
    B.  forked                E.  fused
    C.  cervical                                          A B C D E

4.  Myoblasts from the occipital myotomes are believed to
    give rise to the muscles of the

    A.  eye                   D.  tongue
    B.  ear                   E.  pharynx
    C.  neck                                              A B C D E

5.  The pharyngeal and laryngeal muscles develop from
    mesenchyme derived from the

    A.  preotic myotomes      D.  somatic mesoderm
    B.  occipital myotomes    E.  branchial arches
    C.  splanchnic mesoderm                               A B C D E

6.  Which of the following bones is not derived mainly
    from the cartilaginous viscerocranium?

    A.  Malleus               D.  Occipital
    B.  Incus                 E.  Hyoid
    C.  Stapes                                            A B C D E

7.  Increase in the size of the calvaria ('brain case')
    is greatest during the first _____ years.

    A.  two                   D.  seven
    B.  three                 E.  nine
    C.  five                                              A B C D E

8.  The face of the newborn infant is relatively small compared
    with the calvaria.  Enlargement of the facial region during
    childhood mainly results from an increase in the size of the

    A.  paranasal sinuses
    B.  deciduous teeth
    C.  nose and jaws
    D.  permanent teeth
    E.  brain                                             A B C D E

9.  The skeleton shows clearly on radiographs (x-ray films) by
    the beginning of the _____ week.

    A.  ninth                 D.  thirteenth
    B.  seventh               E.  sixteenth
    C.  eleventh                                          A B C D E

======================= ANSWERS, NOTES, AND EXPLANATIONS =========================

1.  B  The mandible forms almost entirely by intramembranous ossification.  Some endochondral ossification occurs in a small portion of the anterior part of the mandible and at its condyle.  The mesenchyme in the mandibular process of the first branchial arch condenses around the first arch cartilage (Meckel's cartilage) to form a dense fibromembranous tissue; this undergoes intramembranous ossification as the cartilage degenerates.  Hence, endochondral ossification does not occur in Meckel's cartilage as one might expect.

2.  B  The parietal and other flat bones of the neurocranium develop by intramembranous ossification.  The clavicle begins to develop by intramembranous ossification, but later develops growth cartilages at each end which give rise to most of the bone.

3.  A  Lumbar ribs are the most common type of accessory ribs, but they are usually of no clinical significance.  Cervical ribs are attached to the seventh cervical vertebra.  They may be unilateral or bilateral, complete or incomplete.  Usually a cervical rib causes no symptoms; however, the subclavian artery and the inferior part of the branchial plexus may cross over the cervical rib.  In these cases the rib may exert pressure on these structures and give rise to pain and/or muscular atrophy in the upper limb.

4.  D  Initially there are four occipital somites and hence four occipital myotomes.  The first pair of somites disappears and the myotomes of the others give rise to mesenchyme which forms the tongue muscles.  When the myoblasts migrate to the tongue, they carry their nerve supply with them.

5.  E  The mesenchyme that gives rise to the myoblasts that form the pharyngeal and laryngeal muscles, is derived from the fourth and sixth branchial arches.  These muscles are innervated by the vagus nerve (cranial nerve X), the nerve supplying these branchial arches.

6.  D  The occipital bone is mainly derived by ossification of the dorsal part of the cartilaginous neurocranium.  The portion of this bone superior to the highest nuchal line develops by intramembranous ossification.  The cartilaginous viscerocranium consists of the cartilaginous skeleton of the first two pairs of branchial arches.  Parts of the cartilages in these arches undergo endochondral ossification to form bone (e.g., the styloid process of the temporal bone).

7.  A  Growth of the calvaria is very rapid during infancy, especially during the first two years.  This growth is related primarily to the extensive development of the brain during this period.  A person's calvaria normally increases slightly in capacity until 15 or 16 years of age.

8.  A  Enlargement of the frontal and facial regions of the skull results mainly from the increase in size of the paranasal sinuses.  These air sinuses develop during the late fetal period and infancy as small diverticula of the lateral walls of the nasal cavities.  However, during childhood these sinuses also extend into the maxilla, ethmoid, frontal, and sphenoid bones.  This causes enlargement of the face.  There is concurrent development of the jaws

as the teeth develop and erupt.

9. E Although the fetal skeleton may be visualized earlier than sixteen weeks on radiographs, it is usually not clearly displayed until after the fourteenth week. X-ray investigations often raise concerns about the hazards of ionizing radiations. Embryos are particularly radiosensitive during the period of organogenesis. The fetal gonads and the brain are radiosensitive throughout the fetal period. Because of this, ultrasound scans of the uterus are often used to diagnose twins, to locate the placenta, and to study the fetal skull. There is no increased incidence of congenital abnormalities, or evidence of tissue damage caused by sound energy in infants of mothers who have undergone sonography.

# M U L T I - C O M P L E T I O N   Q U E S T I O N S

DIRECTIONS:   In each of the following questions or incomplete statements ONE OR MORE of the completions is correct.  At the lower right of each question, circle A if 1, 2, and 3 are correct; B if 1 and 3 are correct; C if 2 and 4 are correct; D if only 4 is correct; and E if all are correct.

1. Muscles commonly showing variations that are functionally insignificant include:

   1. diaphragm
   2. pectoralis major
   3. abdominal
   4. sternalis            A B C D E

2. Bones that are part of the neurocranium include:

   1. parietal
   2. occipital
   3. frontal
   4. mandible             A B C D E

3. Achondroplasia is

   1. caused by a disturbance of ossification
   2. the most common cause of dwarfism
   3. transmitted as a mendelian dominant
   4. often associated with mental retardation          A B C D E

4. At points where two flat bones of the skull meet, there are:

   1. cartilaginous joints
   2. fontanelles
   3. primary centers
   4. sutures              A B C D E

5. Spina bifida occulata is

   1. usually in the lumbar or sacral region
   2. a bony defect in the vertebral arch
   3. very common and usually asymptomatic
   4. diagnosed by x-ray examination          A B C D E

======================= ANSWERS, NOTES, AND EXPLANATIONS =========================

1. C  2 and 4 are correct.  Absence of the sternocostal part of the pectoralis major muscle is fairly common, and the sternalis muscle is present in only some persons.  These variations are usually functionally insignificant.  Defects of the diaphragm and the anterior abdominal muscles usually result in malformations (e.g., herniation) that require surgical correction.

2. A  1, 2, and 3 are correct.  The parietal and frontal bones are flat bones that form the main part of the membranous neurocranium.  The occipital bone is derived mainly from the cartilaginous neurocranium.  The cartilaginous neurocranium or chondrocranium and the membranous neurocranium together form a protective case for the brain.  The mandible is the largest and strongest bone of the face, but it is not part of the neurocranium.

3. A  1, 2, and 3 are correct.  Mental development is usually normal in persons with achondroplasia.  In this condition, there is imperfect ossification at the epiphyseal cartilage plates of long bones.  Dwarfism results from shortening of the limbs.  The proximal bones are often most affected.  This kind of dwarfism occurs about once in 10,000 newborn infants.

4. D  4 only is correct.  At birth the flat bones are separated from each other by dense connective tissue.  These fibrous joints are called sutures.  At points where three or more bones meet, the sutures are wide and are called fontanelles.  The loose connections of the bones at the sutures enable the skull to undergo changes of shape (e.g., molding during birth).

5. E  All are correct.  This defect in one or more vertebrae results from failure of fusion of the laminae of the vertebral arch.  Spina bifida occulta of the first sacral vertebra occurs in about 10 percent of people.  The abnormality is usually asymptomatic.  Frequently only one vertebra is defective.  Although common, it is usually of no significance.

F I V E - C H O I C E   A S S O C I A T I O N   Q U E S T I O N S

DIRECTIONS:  Each group of questions below consists of a numbered list of descriptive words or phrases accompanied by a diagram with certain parts indicated by letters, or by a list of lettered headings.  For each numbered word or phrase, SELECT THE LETTERED PART OR HEADING that matches it correctly.  Then insert the letter in the space to the right of the appropriate number.  Sometimes more than one numbered word or phrase may be correctly matched to the same lettered part or heading.

A.  Centrum
B.  Epiphyseal plates
C.  Frontal bone
D.  Anterior fontanelle
E.  Cartilaginous
    viscerocranium

1. ____ Closes during the second year
2. ____ Forms by intramembranous ossification
3. ____ Within the first and second branchial arches
4. ____ Growth of long bones
5. ____ A primary ossification center
6. ____ Styloid process

## ASSOCIATION QUESTIONS

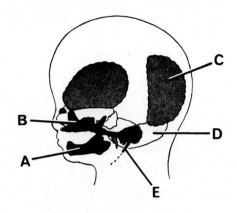

7. _____ Associated with the first branchial arch cartilage
8. _____ Part of the cartilaginous viscerocranium
9. _____ Forms in the maxillary prominence of the first branchial arch
10. _____ Part of the cartilaginous neuro-cranium
11. _____ Forms in the mandibular prominence of the first branchial arch
12. _____ Part of membranous neurocranium

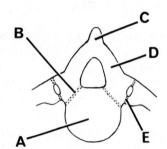

13. _____ Articulates with the centrum
14. _____ Neurocentral joint
15. _____ Replaced by a synovial joint
16. _____ Centrum
17. _____ Disappears during infancy
18. _____ Disappears during childhood

========================= ANSWERS, NOTES, AND EXPLANATIONS =========================

1. D  The anterior fontanelle, located where the two parietal bones and the halves of the frontal bone meet, usually closes about the middle of the second year.  Palpation of this fontanelle during infancy gives information about ossification of the skull and intracranial pressure.

2. C  The frontal bone, part of the membranous neurocranium, develops by intra-membranous ossification from two primary centers.  The halves of the frontal bone begin to fuse during the second year and the frontal or metopic suture is usually obliterated by the eighth year.

3. E  The ends of the cartilaginous rods in the first and second pairs of branchial arches reach the ventral surface of the neurocranium in the region of the developing ears.  Later they undergo endochondral ossification to form

4. B  During the later stages of postnatal bone growth, the mass of cartilage between the diaphysis and epiphysis decreases in thickness to form a comparatively thin cartilage, the epiphyseal cartilage plate. They are of importance for growth of long bones. At the termination of growth in the bone, the epiphyseal plate disappears and the epiphysis unites with the diaphysis.

5. A  Most of the body of a typical vertebra (thoracic and lumbar) is ossified from a primary center, the centrum, which appears during the eighth week. At birth, the bone of the centrum is separated from the separate halves of the vertebral arch of cartilage by the neurocentral joints.

6. E  The styloid process of the temporal bone develops by endochondral ossification of part of the dorsal end of the cartilage of the second branchial arch (Reichert's cartilage). The cartilages of the first two pairs of branchial arches constitute the cartilaginous viscerocranium.

7. A  Development of the mandible is associated with Meckel's cartilage, the cartilage in the mandibular prominence of the first branchial arch. As this cartilage degenerates, the condensed mesenchyme near it undergoes intramembranous ossification to form the mandible (lower jaw).

8. E  The styloid process of the temporal bone, the malleus, incus, and stapes are derived from the cartilaginous viscerocranium (the skeleton of the embryonic jaws).

9. B  The maxilla forms in the maxillary prominence of the first branchial arch by intramembranous ossification. It is a part of the membranous viscerocranium, as are the mandible, zygomatic, and squamous temporal bones.

10. D  The occipital bone ossifies partly by endochondral ossification of the posterior part of the cartilaginous neurocranium. This plate of cartilage forms in the base of the developing skull by the fusion of several paired cartilages.

11. A  The mandible is the part of the membranous viscerocranium which develops mainly by intramembranous ossification around the degenerating cartilage of the first branchial arch.

12. C  The parietal and other flat bones of the skull are parts of the membranous neurocranium, which develop by intramembranous ossification. At birth, they are separated by connective tissue sutures.

13. D  Each half of the vertebral arch, called a lamina, is ossified from a primary ossification center. At birth the halves of the arch are separated from each other dorsally by cartilage, and from the centrum by cartilaginous neurocentral joints. These joints disappear when the vertebral arch fuses with the centrum (usually about the fifth year). The halves of the vertebral arch fuse during the first year; failure of this fusion to occur results in spina bifida occulta.

14. B  As stated above, the neurocentral joints are located between the centrum and the vertebral arch. In the superior cervical vertebrae, the centra unite

with the vertebral arches about the third year, but in the inferior lumbar vertebrae union is not completed until the sixth year.

15. E  The ribs are connected to the costal processes of thoracic vertebrae at costovertebral joints.  As the ribs and vertebrae ossify, joints develop between the tubercles of the ribs and the transverse processes of the vertebrae.

16. A  The major portion of the body of a typical vertebra is formed by the centrum.  It is ossified from a primary center which appears dorsal to the notochord.  The centrum is occasionally ossified from bilateral primary centers.

17. C  The vertebrae form by the ossification of cartilaginous models.  Primary centers appear during the early fetal period: one in each half of the vertebral arch, and one in the centrum.  At birth the ossified halves of the vertebral arch are still separated from each other by cartilage (C).  This cartilage is ossified during the first year.

18. B  The vertebral arch (neural arch) during infancy and early childhood is separated from the bone of the centrum by persistent bilateral zones of cartilage (neurocentral joints).  These two lateral zones are ossified during the fifth or sixth year.

---

NOTES:

# THE LIMBS

## O B J E C T I V E S

BE ABLE TO:

---

- o   Describe the development of the limbs.
- o   Define and illustrate the apical ectodermal ridge.
- o   Describe the development of the bones and muscles of the limbs.
- o   Describe the effects of teratogens on limb development.
- o   Construct and label diagrams illustrating rotation of the limbs.
- o   Discuss and illustrate the development of the dermatomal patterns of the limbs.

---

## F I V E - C H O I C E   C O M P L E T I O N   Q U E S T I O N S

DIRECTIONS:  Each of the following statements or questions is followed by five suggested responses or completions.  SELECT THE ONE BEST ANSWER in each case and then circle the appropriate letter at the right of each question.

1.   Teratogens acting after the _____ week will not cause limb malformations.

A.  fourth
B.  fifth
C.  sixth
D.  seventh
E.  eighth

A B C D E

2.   Each of the following statements about the apical ectodermal ridge is correct except:

A.  It first appears in the upper limb bud.
B.  It exerts an inductive influence on the limb mesenchyme.
C.  It appears at the proximal end of the limb bud.
D.  It promotes growth and development of the limb.
E.  Injury to it results in severe limb defects.

A B C D E

## SELECT THE ONE BEST ANSWER

3.  Each of the following bones is formed mainly by endochondral ossification except:

    A.  humerus            D.  ulna
    B.  hyoid              E.  tibia
    C.  mandible                              A B C D E

4.  Which of the following bones develops by intramembranous ossification?

    A.  humerus            D.  phalanges
    B.  ulna                E.  none of the
    C.  radius                      above        A B C D E

====================== ANSWERS, NOTES, AND EXPLANATIONS ======================

1.  E  By the end of the eighth week, the digits (fingers and toes) are well differentiated; hence after this period, teratogenic substances (e.g., drugs) are unable to produce congenital malformations.

2.  C  The apical ectodermal ridge appears at the distal end of the limb bud. There is strong evidence of inductor activity by the ridge on the mesenchyme in the limb.

3.  C  The mandible forms almost entirely by intramembranous bone formation. The embryonic mandible is supported by the cartilage of the first branchial arch, but it disappears as the mandible develops around it.

4.  E  All the limb bones form by endochondral ossification. Mesenchymal models of the bones form and chondrification results in cartilage models.

## M U L T I - C O M P L E T I O N   Q U E S T I O N S

DIRECTIONS:  In each of the following questions or incomplete statements ONE OR MORE of the completions is correct.  At the lower right of each question, circle A if 1, 2, and 3 are correct; B if 1 and 3 are correct; C if 2 and 4 are correct; D if only 4 is correct; and E if all are correct.

1.  Minor limb defects are relatively common.  Common causes of limb defects at present include:

    1.  mechanical factors       3.  drugs
    2.  thalidomide              4.  genetic factors      A B C D E

| A | B | C | D | E |
|---|---|---|---|---|
| 1,2,3 | 1,3 | 2,4 | only 4 | all correct |

2. Syndactyly is

   1. a relatively common limb malformation
   2. one of the most common hand deformities
   3. more frequent in the foot than in the hand
   4. often caused by hereditary factors                A B C D E

3. During development of the limbs, the

   1. upper limbs rotate laterally
   2. limbs rotate on their axes
   3. lower limbs rotate medially
   4. limbs rotate in the same direction                A B C D E

4. Congenital dislocation of the hip is

   1. much more common in females
   2. associated with hip joint laxity
   3. inherited as a mendelian dominant
   4. associated with underdevelopment of
      the acetabulum                                     A B C D E

5. Correct statements about limb development
   include:

   1. The developing upper limbs originally
      project at a right angle to the body.
   2. The thumb develops on the preaxial border
      of the limb.
   3. The fifth digit of the hand develops on the
      postaxial border of the upper limb.
   4. The lower limb buds differentiate earlier
      than the upper limb buds.                          A B C D E

6. Correct statements about development of the upper
   limbs include:

   1. The limb buds develop opposite the inferior
      two cervical and superior six thoracic
      segments.
   2. The ectoderm at the apices of the upper limb
      buds thickens to form apical ectodermal
      ridges.
   3. During the fourth week, the spinal nerves grow
      into the upper limb buds.
   4. The mesenchymal models of the forearm bones
      undergo chondrification during the sixth week.     A B C D E

| A | B | C | D | E |
|---|---|---|---|---|
| 1,2,3 | 1,3, | 2,4, | only 4 | all correct |

7. The apical ectodermal ridge

   1.  exerts an inductive influence on the loose mesenchyme
      in the limb buds.
   2.  is composed of a thickened layer of surface ectoderm.
   3.  is visible at the apices of the limb buds during the
      fourth week.
   4.  disappears at the end of the fourth week.       A B C D E

8. The limbs

   1.  contain ossification centers in their long bones by
      the 12th week
   2.  arise as buds from the body wall during the fifth week
   3.  develop proximodistally, with the result that the humerus
      is recognizable before the forearm bones
   4.  contain some bones that develop by intramembranous
      ossification       A B C D E

======================= ANSWERS, NOTES, AND EXPLANATIONS =========================

1. D **4 only is correct.** A majority of limb malformations are caused by genetic factors (e.g., chromosomal abnormalities like those in trisomy 18, and mutant genes as in brachydactyly). Between 1957 and 1962, there was an 'epidemic' of limb malformations resulting from maternal ingestion of thalidomide. Since this drug has been withdrawn from the market, major limb malformations are rarely observed. Undoubtedly some malformations result from an interaction of genetic and environmental factors (e.g., congenital dislocation of the hip).

2. E **All are correct.** The fusion of digits can exist in any degree from simple cutaneous webbing to fusion of the bones. Syndactyly may be associated with polydactyly (extra digits) and brachydactyly (short digits). The condition is usually bilateral and is often familial. Simple dominant, or sex-linked dominant, or simple recessive hereditary factors may be involved.

3. A **1, 2, and 3 are correct.** The developing limbs rotate in opposite directions and to different degrees. Hence, the elbows of fetuses point backward, or dorsally, and the knees point forward or ventrolaterally. As a result of the rotations, the extensor muscles come to lie on the external and dorsal aspect of the upper limb, and on the ventral aspect of the lower limb.

4. E **All are correct.** Usually the hip is not fully dislocated at birth. The basic pathology appears to be relaxation of the joint capsule. The condition occurs in about 1 in 1500 infants; one male to 10 females. In Britain, one female in 700 and one male in 5,000 is affected.

5.  A  <u>1, 2, and 3 are correct</u>.  The upper limb buds appear first and differentiate earlier than the lower limb buds.  By the end of the eighth week, the upper and lower limbs are well differentiated.

6.  C  <u>2 and 4 are correct</u>.  The upper limb buds develop opposite the inferior six cervical and the superior two thoracic segments.  The peripheral nerves grow from the brachial plexus into the mesenchyme of the limb buds during the fifth week.

7.  A  <u>1, 2, and 3 are correct</u>.  The ectodermal cells at the tip of each limb multiply during the fourth week to form apical ectodermal ridges.  As the digital rays develop in the sixth week, the apical ectodermal ridges form caps over the distal ends of the digital rays and direct digital development.

8.  B  <u>1 and 3 are correct</u>.  The limb buds are first visible during the fourth week.  The upper limb buds appear at about 26 days and the lower limb buds appear about two days later.  All the bones of the limb develop by endochondral ossification.  This process begins at the end of the embryonic period and ossification centers are present in all the long bones of the limbs by the twelfth week.

F I V E - C H O I C E   A S S O C I A T I O N   Q U E S T I O N S

DIRECTIONS:  Each group of questions below consists of a numbered list of descriptive words or phrases accompanied by a list of lettered headings.  For each numbered word or phrase, SELECT THE LETTERED HEADING that matches it correctly.  Then insert the letter in the space to the right of the appropriate number.  Sometimes more than one numbered word or phrase may be correctly matched to the same lettered heading.

A.  Upper limb buds
B.  Apical ectodermal ridge
C.  Somatic mesoderm
D.  Meromelia
E.  Lower limb buds

1. ____  Partial absence of a limb
2. ____  Limb muscles
3. ____  Rotate medially
4. ____  Rotate laterally
5. ____  Exerts an inductive influence
6. ____  Thalidomide ingestion

A.  Dermatome
B.  Phocomelia
C.  Digital rays
D.  End of fourth week
E.  Amelia

7. ____  Condensations of mesenchyme
8. ____  Lower limb bud develops
9. ____  Area of skin supplied by a
         spinal nerve
10. ____  Absence of the limbs
11. ____  A type of meromelia

======================= ANSWERS, NOTES, AND EXPLANATIONS =========================

1.  D  Meromelia (from Greek meros, 'part' and melos, 'extremity') is the term now used to classify all limb malformations involving partial absence of a limb or limbs, e.g., hemimelia (absence of all or part of the distal half of a limb), and phocomelia (absence of the proximal part of a limb or limbs).

2.  C  The limb muscles develop from mesenchyme that is derived from the somatic mesoderm.  Hence, the musculature develops in situ and is not derived from mesenchyme in the myotome regions of the somites.

3.  E  The developing lower limbs rotate medially through almost 90 degrees.  As a result, the knees face anterolaterally.

4.  A  The developing upper limbs rotate laterally through 90 degrees on their longitudinal axes; as a result, the elbows face dorsally or posteriorly.

5.  B  The apical ectodermal ridge is a thickened, epithelial plaque at the distal end of each limb bud.  This ridge is an inducer of limb growth.  There is no further elaboration of distal structures (hands and fingers) if the ridge is removed experimentally.

6.  D  Meromelia or partial absence of the limbs was commonly observed in the infants of mothers who ingested thalidomide during the critical period of limb development (4th - 6th weeks of development).

7.  C  The digital rays are condensations of mesenchyme in the hand and foot plates which indicate where the digits will develop.

8.  D  The lower limb buds appear at the end of the fourth week as ventro-lateral outgrowths of the body wall.

9.  A  A dermatome is the area of skin supplied by a single spinal nerve and its spinal ganglion (dorsal root ganglion).

10. E  Amelia refers to absence of the limbs.  This condition resulted when thalidomide was ingested by pregnant women early in the fourth week after fertilization.

11. B  Phocomelia is a type of meromelia (partial absence of the limbs).  In this type of meromelia, the limbs have a flipper-like appearance.

---

NOTES:

# THE NERVOUS SYSTEM

## O B J E C T I V E S

BE ABLE TO:

---

o   Construct and label diagrams showing early development of the nervous system.

o   Define the following: neural plate, neural groove, neural folds, neural crest, neuropores, primary and secondary brain vesicles.

o   Make a simple diagram illustrating the development of neurons and neuroglial cells.

o   Construct and label diagrams illustrating the brain flexures and indicating the adult derivatives of the walls and cavities of the forebrain, midbrain, and hindbrain.

o   Prepare sketches illustrating the development of the hypophysis cerebri (pituitary gland).

o   Discuss the following congenital malformations of the central nervous system, using sketches as required: meroanencephaly, microcephaly, encephalocele, cranial meningocele, Arnold-Chiari malformation, spina bifida with meningocele, and spina bifida with meningomyelocele.

---

## F I V E - C H O I C E   C O M P L E T I O N   Q U E S T I O N S

DIRECTIONS: Each of the following statements or questions is followed by five suggested responses or completions. SELECT THE ONE BEST ANSWER in each case and then circle the appropriate letter at the right of each question.

1.   The rostral and caudal neuropores usually close during the _____ week.

   A.  third                    D.  sixth
   B.  fourth                   E.  seventh
   C.  fifth                                            A B C D E

2.   The pons and cerebellum are derived from the walls of the

   A.  hindbrain                D.  midbrain
   B.  mesencephalon            E.  metencephalon
   C.  myelencephalon                                   A B C D E

3. The myelin sheaths surrounding axons in the central nervous system are formed by

    A. neuroglial cells
    B. astrocytes
    C. oligodendrocytes

    D. microglial cells
    E. Schwann cells

    A B C D E

4. Each of the following cells in the central nervous system is derived from neuroepithelial cells except:

    A. ependymal cells
    B. microglial cells
    C. astroglia

    D. motor neurons
    E. choroid epithelial cells

    A B C D E

5. Each of the following cells is derived from the neural crest except:

    A. melanocyte
    B. Schwann cell
    C. ependymal cell

    D. chromaffin cell
    E. spinal ganglion cell

    A B C D E

6. The brain flexure which develops between the metencephalon and the myelencephalon is called the ____ flexure.

    A. pontine
    B. cervical
    C. hindbrain

    D. midbrain
    E. cerebellar

    A B C D E

7. The neurolemma and myelin sheath of a peripheral nerve fiber are formed by

    A. mesenchymal cells
    B. microglia
    C. neural cells

    D. Schwann cells
    E. neuroepithelial cells

    A B C D E

8. The longitudinal groove in the internal surface of the developing spinal cord is called the

    A. neural groove
    B. cuneate groove
    C. sulcus limitans

    D. sulcus longitudinalis
    E. longitudinal groove

    A B C D E

9. Each of the following is a derivative of the alar plates except:

    A. gracile nucleus
    B. pontine nucleus
    C. dorsal gray horn

    D. cuneate nucleus
    E. ventral gray horn

    A B C D E

SELECT THE ONE BEST ANSWER

10. Which of the following structures is <u>not</u> a derivative of the diencephalon?

    A. thalamus
    B. adenohypophysis
    C. hypothalamus
    D. neurohypophysis
    E. epithalamus

    A B C D E

11. The formation of myelin sheaths is largely completed by the end of the ____ period.

    A. embryonic
    B. fetal
    C. perinatal
    D. neonatal
    E. infantile

    A B C D E

12. The pineal body develops as a diverticulum of the roof of the

    A. telencephalon
    B. diencephalon
    C. forebrain
    D. mesencephalon
    E. midbrain

    A B C D E

13. At birth the caudal end of the spinal cord lies at the level of the ____ ____ vertebra.

    A. third sacral
    B. first sacral
    C. third lumbar
    D. first lumbar
    E. twelfth thoracic

    A B C D E

14. Which of the following may follow infection with cytomegalovirus or <u>Toxoplasma</u> <u>gondii</u> during the fetal period?

    A. mental retardation
    B. hydrocephaly
    C. microcephaly
    D. microphthalmia
    E. all of the above

    A B C D E

15. Which of the following congenital abnormalities of the central nervous system is illustrated?

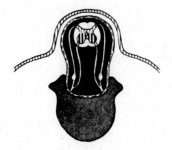

    A. Spina bifidia with meningocele
    B. Spina bifida cystica
    C. Spina bifida occulta
    D. Spina bifida with myeloschisis
    E. Spina bifida with meningomyelocele

    A B C D E

======================= ANSWERS, NOTES, AND EXPLANATIONS ==========================

1.  B  The cranial opening in the neural tube, called the rostral neuropore, closes at about 26 days and the caudal neuropore closes about two days later. Failure of the neural folds to fuse and form the forebrain vesicle, or failure of the rostral neuropore to close results in meroanencephaly (anencephaly). The brain is represented by a mass of largely degenerated nervous tissue. Failure of the neural folds to fuse into the neural tube in the region that gives rise to the spinal cord, or failure of the caudal neuropore to close, results in spina bifida cystica (e.g., spina bifida with meningocele).

2.  E  The walls of the metencephalon give rise to the pons and cerebellum; its cavity forms the superior part of the fourth ventricle. If you chose answer A, you were partly correct because the metencephalon is the rostal part of the hindbrain. Answer E is more specific; thus it is the best answer.

3.  C  The oligodendrocytes are responsible for the formation of myelin sheaths in the central nervous system in the same way that Schwann cells form the myelin sheaths of peripheral nerve fibers. The plasma membrane of an oligodendrocyte becomes wrapped around a fiber. The number of layers that are wrapped around the fiber determines the thickness of the myelin sheath. If you selected choice A, you were partly right because oligodendrocytes are a type of neuroglial cell. However, choice C is more specific; thus it is the best answer.

4.  B  The microglial cells (microglia), scattered through the gray and white matter of the central nervous system, are derived from mesoderm. They invade the central nervous system late in fetal development. To indicate their mesodermal origin, this type of neuroglial cell is sometimes called a mesoglial cell.

5.  C  Ependymal cells, often classified as a type of neuroglial cell, are derived from the neuroepithelium of the neural tube. After the production of neuroblasts (developing neurons) has ceased, the neuroepithelial cells lining the ventricles and the central canal of the spinal cord form the ependymal epithelium or ependyma. Throughout most of the ventricular surface, the ependymal cells have cilia which project into the ventricles. The ependyma that covers the capillaries of the choroid plexuses is of the cuboidal type and is called the choroid plexus epithelium.

6.  A  The pontine flexure causes the lateral walls of the medulla to fall outward or laterally like the pages of an opening book. This causes the roof plate to become stretched and the cavity of the hindbrain (future fourth ventricle) to become somewhat rhomboidal or diamond-shaped.

7.  D  The neurolemma and myelin sheath are both components of Schwann cells derived from the neural crest. These cells migrate peripherally and wrap themselves around the fibers of peripheral nerves. One Schwann cell may envelop up to 15 fibers which remain as unmyelinated fibers. Schwann cells ensheathing a single axon develop myelin between the axon and the neurolemma by rotation of the Schwann cell around the axon.

8.  C  The sulcus limitans results from differential thickening of the lateral walls of the developing spinal cord. This sulcus or groove demarcates the dorsal or alar plate (lamina) from the ventral or basal plate (lamina). This regional separation is of fundamental importance because the alar and basal plates are later associated with afferent and efferent functions respectively.

9.  E  The neurons forming the gray matter in the ventral (anterior) horns of the spinal cord are derived from neuroblasts in the basal plates. The lateral gray columns of the spinal cord are also derived from the basal plates. The alar laminae form the gray columns in the dorsal horns.

10. B  The adenohypophysis or glandular portion of the hypophysis or pituitary gland is not derived from the diencephalon. It originates from Rathke's pouch, a diverticulum from the roof of the primitive mouth or stomodeum. The neurohypophysis is derived from the infundibulum, a downgrowth from the floor of the diencephalon.

11. E  Myelination begins during midfetal life (16 to 20 weeks) and is largely completed by the end of the infantile period (12-14 months). There are exceptions to these general statements, e.g., the descending motor tracts (pyramidal and rubrospinal) do not begin to acquire their myelin sheaths until full term, and the process is not complete until the end of the second year of postnatal life. There is good evidence to indicate that tracts become completely myelinated at about the time they become fully functional.

12. B  The pineal body (gland), also called the epiphysis, develops as a midline diverticulum of the caudal part of the roof of the diencephalon. Eventually it becomes a solid organ located on the roof of the mesencephalon (midbrain). When stimulated, sympathetic fibers in the pineal body release norepinephrine.

13. C  The caudal or inferior end of the spinal cord usually lies at the level of the third lumbar vertebra in the newborn. This is an average level; it could end as high as the second lumbar vertebra or as low as the fourth lumbar vertebra. In the embryo the spinal cord extends the entire length of the vertebral canal. However, because the vertebral column grows more rapidly than the spinal cord, the cord gradually comes to lie at relatively higher levels. Because a portion of the subarachnoid space extends below the spinal cord (i.e., below $L_3$ in the newborn), cerebrospinal fluid may be removed without damaging the cord. In the adult, the spinal cord usually ends at the inferior border of the first lumbar vertebra.

14. E  Maternal infections (cytomegalovirus and Toxoplasma gondii) during the fetal period may cause all the congenital abnormalities listed. Rubella infections during the second trimester often produce effects similar to those caused by cytomegalovirus and the parasite Toxoplasma gondii, except that the rubella virus usually causes more severe abnormalities, especially of the eyes and ears.

15. E  If you chose B, you selected the second best answer; it is not as specific as choice E because A and D are also types of spina bifida cystica, i.e., they exhibit a saccular protrusion of the spinal cord and/or the meninges.

# M U L T I - C O M P L E T I O N   Q U E S T I O N S

DIRECTIONS: In each of the following questions or incomplete statements ONE OR MORE of the completions is correct. At the lower right of each question, circle A if 1, 2, and 3 are correct; B if 1 and 3 are correct; C if 2 and 4 are correct; D if only 4 is correct; and E if all are correct.

1. In which of the following congenital malformations is there usually no neurological involvement?

   1. spina bifida with meningocele    3. spina bifida cystica
   2. spina bifida with myeloschisis    4. spina bifida occulta      A B C D E

2. The Schwann cells give rise to the

   1. endoneurium            3. perineurium
   2. neurolemma             4. myelin sheath        A B C D E

3. Cells differentiating from neural crest cells include:

   1. sympathetic ganglion cell    3. satellite cells
   2. spinal ganglion cell        4. chromaffin cells     A B C D E

4. Spina bifida cystica commonly occurs in which of the following regions?

   1. lower thoracic         3. sacral
   2. lumbar                4. coccygeal         A B C D E

5. Conditions often associated with spina bifida cystica include:

   1. hydrocephalus         3. nerve involvement
   2. muscle paralysis       4. loss of sensation    A B C D E

6. Malformations often associated with spina bifida with meningomyelocele include:

   1. Arnold-Chiari malformation    3. clubfoot
   2. vertebral defects        4. amyelia           A B C D E

7. Causes of excess cerebrospinal fluid (CSF) or hydrocephalus that are the most likely basis for this condition during infancy include:

   1. overproduction of CSF
   2. defective absorption of CSF
   3. failure of absorption of CSF
   4. obstruction to CSF circulation          A B C D E

| A | B | C | D | E |
|---|---|---|---|---|
| 1,2,3 | 1,3 | 2,4 | only 4 | all correct |

8. Congenital internal hydrocephalus usually results from atresia of the

   1. cerebral aqueduct
   2. foramina of Monro
   3. foramen of Magendie
   4. foramina of Luschka                    A B C D E

9. The walls of the hindbrain vesicle give rise to the

   1. pons                    3. medulla oblongata
   2. cerebellum              4. pyramids        A B C D E

10. Mental retardation may result from

   1. chromosomal abnormalities    3. fetal infections
   2. metabolic disturbances       4. irradiation    A B C D E


======================= ANSWERS, NOTES, AND EXPLANATIONS =========================


1. D **4 only is correct**. Spina bifida occulta is the most common variety of spina bifida and the least serious type. This is a defect of the vertebral column which results from failure of fusion of the halves of the vertebral arch in one or more vertebrae. Spina bifida occulta usually occurs in the sacrolumbar region and is covered by skin. The spinal cord and nerves are usually normal. The other types of spina bifida listed show varying degrees of neurological involvement, depending on the position and the extent of the lesion. The level of the lesion determines the area of anesthesia and which muscles are affected.

2. C **2 and 4 are correct**. The neurolemma and the myelin sheath are both derivatives of Schwann cells. The Schwann cells are responsible for laying down the myelin sheath around the axis cylinder. Electron microscopic studies have shown that the myelin is not only formed by the Schwann cell, but consists of its plasma membrane wrapped around the axis cylinder. The term neurolemmal sheath (neurolemma) or sheath of Schwann is used to distinguish the nucleated cytoplasmic layer from the layer of myelin. The connective tissue layers (endoneurium, perineurium and epineurium) are derived from mesenchyme.

3. E **All are correct**. The peripheral nervous system is derived in part from cells from the neural tube which give rise to the motor nerve fibers of the spinal and cranial nerves. The afferent neurons of the peripheral and autonomic nervous systems are almost all derived from the neural crest. There is also evidence that neural crest cells give rise to mesenchymal cells in the head region.

4.  A  <u>1, 2, and 3 are correct</u>.  Nonfusion of the vertebral laminae associated with meningocele or myelomeningocele commonly occurs in the first three regions listed but is not common in the coccygeal region.  Meningomyeloceles are occasionally observed in the sacrococcygeal region.  In more than half of the cases of spina bifida cystica, the defect is located in the lumbar region.

5.  E  <u>All are correct</u>.  A large proportion of meningomyeloceles are associated with hydrocephalus.  Often there are associated malformations of the cerebral aqueduct of the midbrain.  Often the hydrocephalus is not obvious at birth, but in most cases is diagnosed by three months of age.  Though the spinal cord may be in the normal position, abnormalities of it may exist, resulting in nerve and skeletal muscle involvement.  There may be severe paralysis of the lower limbs, involvement of the bladder and anal sphincters, and loss of sensation (often in the buttocks, perineum and medial aspects of the thighs, producing the so-called saddle anesthesia).

6.  A  <u>1, 2, and 3 are correct</u>.  Amyelia (total absence of the spinal cord) is found only in association with meroanencephaly (anencephaly).  Vertebral defects (nonfusion of the vertebral laminae) are present in all cases of spina bifida, as the term indicates.  Abnormalities of the vertebral bodies may lead to kyphosis or scoliosis.  The talipes equinovarus type of clubfoot is very frequently associated with spina bifida with meningomyelocele.  Nearly all myeloceles, except those located inferiorly, have an Arnold-Chiari malformation.

7.  D  <u>4 only is correct</u>.  In all cases of hydrocephalus there is an excess of cerebrospinal fluid (CSF)  Obstruction to the CSF pathway is pathologically and numerically the most important cause of hydrocephalus.  In infants, the excess fluid is usually in the ventricles, resulting in their dilation; one or all the ventricles may be enlarged.  In external hydrocephalus, the excess fluid is mainly in the subarachnoid space.

8.  B  <u>1 and 3 are correct</u>.  Obstruction of the flow of cerebrospinal fluid by atresia (occlusion) of the cerebral aqueduct is the common cause of internal hydrocephalus (dilatation of the ventricles).  It is unlikely that hydrocephalus would result from atresia of the foramina of Luschka; however, if both the median and lateral apertures of the fourth ventricle (foramina of Magendie and Luschka) were occluded, all the ventricles would be enlarged.  Very rarely, one or both ventricles are enlarged because of occlusion of one or both of the interventricular foramina (of Monro).

9.  A  <u>1, 2, and 3 are correct</u>.  Corticospinal fibers from the developing cerebral cortex pass through the ventral part of the wall of the hindbrain, and eventually form a pair of fiber bundles called the pyramids.  Hence, the pyramids develop in the walls of the hindbrain, but they are not derivatives of the walls of the hindbrain.

10.  E  <u>All are correct</u>.  Congenital impairment of intelligence may result from various genetic factors (e.g., numerical and structural chromosomal abnormalities, and mutant genes).  Environmental factors (e.g., rubella, cytomegalovirus, and <u>Toxoplasma gondii</u> infections, drugs, lack of iodine, and ionizing

radiations) are known causes of mental retardation.  A large number of inborn errors of metabolism, resulting from defective gene action (e.g., phenylketonuria), are frequently accompanied by or cause various degrees of mental retardation.


F I V E - C H O I C E   A S S O C I A T I O N   Q U E S T I O N S


DIRECTIONS:  Each group of questions below consists of a numbered list of descriptive words or phrases accompanied by a diagram with certain parts indicated by letters, or by a list of lettered headings.  For each numbered word or phrase, SELECT THE LETTERED PART OR HEADING that matches it correctly.  Then insert the letter in the space to the right of the appropriate number.  Sometimes more than one numbered word or phrase may be correctly matched to the same lettered part or heading.

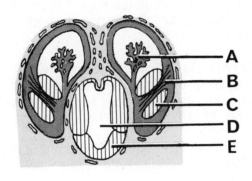

1. ____ Lentiform nucleus
2. ____ An invagination of pia mater
3. ____ Third ventricle
4. ____ Produces cerebrospinal fluid
5. ____ Hypothalamus
6. ____ Internal capsule

A.  Neural crest cells
B.  Alar plates
C.  Basal plates
D.  Neuroepithelium
E.  Spinal ganglion cells

7. ____ Gracile nuclei
8. ____ Form ventral gray columns
9. ____ Sympathetic ganglion cells
10. ____ Neuroglia
11. ____ Efferent function
12. ____ Unipolar afferent neurons

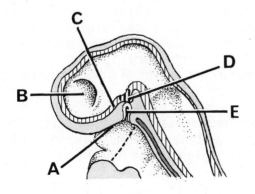

13. ____ Primordium of adenohypophysis
14. ____ Gives rise to the pars nervosa
15. ____ Roof of primitive mouth cavity
16. ____ Infundibulum
17. ____ Primordium of the cerebral hemisphere
18. ____ Floor of the diencephalon

## ASSOCIATION QUESTIONS

A. Telencephalon
B. Diencephalon
C. Mesencephalon
D. Metencephalon
E. Myelencephalon

19. ____ Pons
20. ____ Olivary nuclei
21. ____ Corpus striatum
22. ____ Thalamus
23. ____ Red nuclei
24. ____ Cerebellum
25. ____ Neurohypophyseal bud

======================== ANSWERS, NOTES, AND EXPLANATIONS ========================

1. C  As the cerebral cortex differentiates, nerve fibers passing to and from it pass through the swelling called the corpus striatum in the floor of each hemisphere.  Soon these fibers divide the corpus striatum into two groups of nerve cells, the caudate and lentiform nuclei.

2. A  The choroid plexus of the lateral ventricle is formed by an invagination of vascular pia mater, called the tela choroidea, on the medial side of each cerebral hemisphere.  The vascular connective tissue acquires a covering layer of epithelium from the ependymal lining of the ventricle.

3. D  The third ventricle is formed mainly from the cavity of the diencephalon. The extreme anterior part of the third ventricle is derived from the cavity of the telencephalon.

4. A  The choroid plexuses of the lateral, third, and fourth ventricles produce most of the cerebrospinal fluid (CSF).  The plexuses in the lateral ventricles are the largest and most important producers of CSF.  Some CSF is formed by the pia mater on the external surface of the brain.

5. E  The hypothalamus arises by proliferation of neuroblasts in the ventral wall of the diencephalon.  The various nuclei which develop in it are concerned with endocrine activities and homeostasis.

6. B  As the cerebral cortex differentiates, fibers passing to and from it pass through the corpus striatum; this fiber pathway is called the internal capsule.  Projection fibers concentrated in the internal capsule fan out to form the corona radiata in the medullary center.  Because of its adaptation to the contours of the masses of gray matter in the brain, the internal capsule develops an anterior limb, a genu, and a posterior limb, as seen on horizontal section.

7. B  The gracile and cuneate nuclei develop from neuroblasts that migrate from the alar plates into the marginal zone of the myelencephalon.  These nuclei are associated with correspondingly named tracts which enter the medulla from the spinal cord.

8.  C  The basal plates of the neural tube give rise to the ventral and lateral gray columns of nerve cells in the spinal cord. Axons of the ventral horn cells grow out of the spinal cord and form the ventral roots of spinal nerves.

9.  A  Sympathetic ganglion cells are derived from neuroblasts which differentiate from neural crest cells. Some sympathetic neuroblasts migrate to the suprarenal (adrenal) glands where they differentiate into chromaffin cells of the suprarenal medulla.

10. D  Some neuroepithelial cells of the neural tube differentiate into glioblasts (also called spongioblasts). These cells give rise to oligodendroblasts and astroblasts which eventually become oligodendrocytes and astrocytes. Oligodendrocytes are concerned with the formation of myelin sheaths within the central nervous system and astrocytes provide nutrition and general support to the developing neurons. The formation of glial cells continues into adult life.

11. C  Neuroepithelial cells in the basal plates of the developing neural tube give rise to neurons (e.g., the motor neurons in the ventral horns of the spinal cord) that are concerned with efferent activities.

12. E  The unipolar spinal (dorsal root) ganglion cells arise by differentiation of neural crest cells. First bipolar neuroblasts form and then their processes unite to form unipolar neurons. The central process of this T-shaped axon grows into the spinal cord to form part of a dorsal root; the peripheral process forms part of the dorsal root which joins the ventral root to form a mixed spinal nerve.

13. E  The primordium of the adenohypophysis is Rathke's pouch, a diverticulum from the ectodermal roof of the primitive mouth cavity or stomodeum. This diverticulum grows toward the brain and soon contacts the infundibulum, the primordium of the neurohypophysis.

14. D  The infundibulum gives rise to the neurohypophysis. The infundibulum appears as a ventral bud or diverticulum of the floor of the diencephalon. Later nerve fibers from the hypothalamus grow into the developing pars nervosa of the pituitary gland.

15. A  The epithelial roof of the primitive mouth cavity or stomodeum is derived from ectoderm. As the head folds and the branchial arches form during the fourth week, the surface ectoderm becomes depressed to form the primitive mouth cavity in the center of the facial primordia. Rathke's pouch develops as a dorsal diverticulum of this oral ectoderm.

16. D  The infundibulum, as previously stated, gives rise to the neurohypophysis or pars nervosa of the hypophysis or pituitary gland. As the posterior pituitary develops, the neuroepithelial cells in the wall of the infundibulum proliferate and differentiate into pituicytes.

17. B  The lateral diverticulum of the telencephalon, indicated in the drawing, gives rise to the right cerebral hemisphere. As it expands, it covers the

diencephalon, midbrain, and hindbrain. It eventually meets the other hemisphere in the midline, flattening their medial surfaces.

18. C  The floor of the diencephalon gives rise to the infundibulum (the primordium of the neurohypophysis) and to the mammillary bodies. The infundibulum gives rise to the median eminence, the infundibular stem and the pars nervosa. Initially the infundibulum has a thin wall, but its distal end soon becomes thickened as the neuroepithelial cells proliferate. These cells later differentiate into pituicytes.

19. D  The pons is derived from the metencephalon. Nerve fibers connecting the cerebral and cerebellar cortices with the spinal cord, pass through the marginal layer of the ventral region of the metencephalon. These fibers form a robust band of nerve fibers crossing to the other side. This accounts for the name pons, which is a Latin word meaning 'bridge'. The walls of the metencephalon form the pons and cerebellum, and its cavity forms the superior part of the fourth ventricle.

20. E  The olivary nuclei in the rostral part of the myelencephalon ('open' part of the medulla) are derived from neuroblasts which migrate from the alar plates.

21. A  The corpus striatum appears as a prominent swelling in the floor of each cerebral hemisphere. The hemispheres develop from lateral diverticula of telencephalon. Because of the presence of the corpus striatum in the floor of the hemisphere, the floor expands more slowly than the thin cortical walls. Consequently, the cerebral hemispheres assume a C-shape.

22. B  The thalamus develops from a swelling on each side of the lateral wall of the diencephalon. As the thalamic swellings enlarge, they bulge into the cavity of the diencephalon (developing third ventricle) reducing it to a narrow cavity. The thalamic swellings often meet and fuse in the midline, forming the interthalamic connexus (massa intermedia) which bridges the cavity of the third ventricle.

23. C  The red nuclei of the midbrain are derived from neuroblasts that arise from the basal plates of the mesencephalon. The basal plates also give rise to the nuclei of the third and fourth cranial nerves, and neurons of the reticular nuclei.

24. D  The cerebellum develops from symmetrical thickenings of the rostrodorsal parts of the alar plates of the metencephalon. The cerebellar swellings bulge into the cavity of the metencephalon (future fourth ventricle). Eventually these primordia fuse and overgrow the rostral half of the fourth ventricle and overlap the pons and the medulla.

25. B  The neurohypophyseal bud develops as a ventral diverticulum of the floor of the diencephalon. This bud enlarges to form the infundibulum, the primordium of the median eminence, the infundibular stem, and the pars nervosa of the pituitary gland.

# THE EYE AND EAR

## O B J E C T I V E S

BE ABLE TO:

o   Construct and label diagrams showing early development of the eyes.

o   Define optic sulci, optic vesicles, optic stalks, optic fissures, optic cups, lens placodes, lens pits, and lens vesicles.

o   Describe the development of the retina, ciliary body, and iris, using labelled sketches.

o   Write brief notes on the formation of the lens, choroid, sclera, cornea, and optic nerve.

o   Construct and label diagrams showing the development of the internal ear, middle ear, and external ear.

o   Define otic placode, otic pit, otic vesicle, endolymphatic duct and sac, spiral organ (of Corti), and semicircular ducts.

o   Discuss the embryological basis of the following congenital malformations: coloboma, glaucoma, cataract, and deafness.

## F I V E - C H O I C E   C O M P L E T I O N   Q U E S T I O N S

DIRECTIONS: Each of the following statements or questions is followed by five suggested responses or completions. SELECT THE ONE BEST ANSWER in each case and then circle the appropriate letter at the right of each question.

1.  Which of the following structures is <u>not</u> derived from neuro-ectoderm?

   A.  Epithelium of the iris       D.  Muscles of the iris
   B.  Optic nerve               E.  Retina
   C.  Corneal epithelium                         A B C D E

2.  Which of the following structures is <u>not</u> derived from mesoderm?

   A.  Choroid                D.  Membranous labyrinth
   B.  Bony labyrinth          E.  Sclera
   C.  Extrinsic eye muscles                   A B C D E

## SELECT THE ONE BEST ANSWER

3. Structures derived from the surface ectoderm include the

   A. lens
   B. otic vesicle
   C. external acoustic meatus
   D. corneal epithelium
   E. all of the above

   A B C D E

4. The epithelium of the iris develops from the

   A. inner layer of the rim of the optic cup
   B. outer layer of the rim of the optic cup
   C. both layers of the rim of the optic cup
   D. mesenchyme near the rim of the optic cup
   E. mesenchyme between the lens and the cornea

   A B C D E

5. The inner, nonpigmented portion of the ciliary epithelium is continuous with the

   A. neural layer of the retina
   B. sphincter of the pupil
   C. pigmented epithelium of the retina
   D. anterior surface of the iris
   E. corneal epithelium

   A B C D E

6. The choroid is derived from the

   A. mesoderm surrounding the eye primordium
   B. loose mesenchyme near the optic cup
   C. mesenchyme from the occipital myotomes
   D. mesenchyme between the developing sclera
      and the pigmented layer of the retina
   E. mesenchyme from the first pair of bran-
      chial arches

   A B C D E

7. Cellular components of the retina derived from the inner layer of the optic cup include:

   A. rod cells
   B. ganglion cells
   C. neuroglial cells
   D. bipolar cells
   E. all of the above

   A B C D E

8. During examination of the eyes of a newborn, you noted that one pupil was pear-shaped owing to a defect in the iris. What is the most likely cause of this typical coloboma of the iris?

   A. Genetic factors
   B. Rubella virus
   C. Toxoplasmosis
   D. Radiation
   E. Cytomegalovirus

   A B C D E

SELECT THE ONE BEST ANSWER

9.  You examine a newborn infant and diagnose congenital heart disease. You also observe bilateral cataracts. During discussions with the infant's mother, you learn that she had a fever, sore throat, and a rash on her face, body, and limbs shortly after her first missed period. She also recalled taking some tranquilizers and sedatives during early pregnancy to settle her nerves and to help her sleep. What do you think would be the most likely cause of the congenital malformations you have detected in her baby?

    A.  Measles (rubeola)
    B.  Congenital galactosemia
    C.  Teratogenic drugs
    D.  Influenza
    E.  None of the above

    A B C D E

10. The otic vesicle or otocyst gives rise to the

    A.  saccule
    B.  utricle
    C.  cochlear duct
    D.  endolymphatic sac
    E.  all of the above

    A B C D E

======================= ANSWERS, NOTES, AND EXPLANATIONS =========================

1.  C  The cornea has a dual origin: the stratified squamous, nonkeratinizing epithelium is derived from the surface ectoderm; the substantia propria and other parts of the cornea are derived from mesoderm. Usually muscles are derived from mesoderm. However, the dilator and sphincter pupillae muscles of the iris are exceptions. They are derived from the neuroectoderm of the outer layer of the optic cup.

2.  D  The membranous labyrinth is derived from the otic vesicle (otocyst) which develops from an invagination of the surface ectoderm. The otic vesicle soon loses its connection with the surface (future skin).

3.  E  All these structures are derived from the surface ectoderm. The lens develops from the lens vesicle; the otic vesicle gives rise to the membranous labyrinth; the external acoustic meatus develops from the first branchial groove, and the corneal epithelium arises directly from the surface ectoderm. Other parts of the cornea are derived from mesoderm.

4.  C  The double-layered, pigmented epithelium of the iris develops from the inner and outer layers of the rim of the optic cup. Because this epithelium is continuous with the ciliary epithelium and the retina, it is often wrongly assumed to be homologous only to the pigmented layers of these structures derived from the outer layer of the optic cup.

5.  A  The ciliary epithelium is composed of two layers of cells derived from the ventral continuation of the two layers of the retina. The cells of the inner, nonpigmented portion of the ciliary epithelium are continuous with the

neural layer of the retina. However, they become heavily pigmented in the iridial portion of the retina.

6.  D  Three of these answers are correct, (A,B, and D), but D is the best answer because it is most specific. The mesenchyme surrounding the optic cup differentiates into an inner vascular layer, the choroid, and an outer fibrous layer, the sclera.

7.  E  All these cells are derived from the inner layer of the optic cup. The rod photoreceptor cells are more numerous than the cone photoreceptors. The bipolar cells are true neurons interposed between the photoreceptor cells and the ganglion cells. The inner layers of the retina, in particular, contain neuroglial cells similar to those in the gray matter of the brain.

8.  A  Most cases of coloboma of the iris are genetically determined with dominant transmission. Some colobomas are associated with maternal infections (including rubella and toxoplasmosis), and it is possible that these and other teratogenic factors may produce colobomas because development of colobomas can be induced experimentally in animals. The embryological basis of a typical coloboma of the iris is failure of the optic fissure on the inferior surface of the optic cup to close. Normally closure of this fissure occurs during the sixth week.

9.  E  None of the factors listed likely caused the malformations exhibited by the infant. The most likely cause of these abnormalities was maternal rubella (German measles) during early pregnancy. The infant exhibited two of the common abnormalities of the <u>congenital rubella syndrome</u> (congenital heart disease and cataracts). Though congenital galactosemia could cause the cataracts, this is an uncommon cause. Tranquilizers are not known to cause malformations and thalidomide is the only sedative known to be teratogenic. Influenza and rubeola are not known to be causes of congenital malformations.

10. E  All these structures are derived from the otic vesicle (otocyst), derived from the surface ectoderm. The cochlear duct contains the spiral organ (of Corti), the receptor of auditory stimuli. The other parts of the membranous labyrinth, derived from the otic vesicle, contain sensory areas of the vestibular system.

## M U L T I - C O M P L E T I O N   Q U E S T I O N S

DIRECTIONS:  In each of the following questions or incomplete statements ONE OR MORE of the completions is correct. At the lower right of each question, circle <u>A if 1, 2, and 3</u> are correct; <u>B if 1 and 3</u> are correct; <u>C if 2 and 4</u> are correct; <u>D if only 4</u> is correct; and <u>E if all</u> are correct.

1.  The eyes are derived from the

    1.  surface ectoderm          3.  neuroectoderm
    2.  mesoderm                  4.  first pharyngeal pouch          A B C D E

| A | B | C | D | E |
|---|---|---|---|---|
| 1,2,3 | 1,3 | 2,4 | only 4 | all correct |

2. The middle ear bones or auditory ossicles develop

   1. from the mesenchyme surrounding the tympanic cavity
   2. from the dorsal ends of the first and second
      branchial arch cartilages
   3. by intramembranous ossification
   4. by endochondral ossification             A B C D E

3. Parts of the auditory system are derived from the

   1. endoderm           3. first branchial groove
   2. mesoderm          4. first pharyngeal pouch   A B C D E

4. Structures derived from the neuroectoderm include:

   1. corneal epithelium    3. lens
   2. iris muscles        4. retina            A B C D E

5. Structures derived from the surface ectoderm include:

   1. cochlear duct       3. corneal epithelium
   2. choroid           4. modiolus         A B C D E

6. Parts of the auditory system derived from the otic vesicle
include:

   1. tympanic membrane   3. auricle (pinna)
   2. basilar membrane    4. spiral organ     A B C D E

7. True statements about congenital cataracts include:

   1. Cataracts are relatively common lens malformations.
   2. These lens opacities are usually bilateral.
   3. Some cataracts are genetically determined.
   4. Maternal infections are a common cause.     A B C D E

8. Congenital ocular malformations resulting from absence or
incomplete development of the sinus venosus sclerae or
canal of Schlemm include:

   1. megalocornea      3. ectopia lentis
   2. coloboma         4. glaucoma         A B C D E

9. Types of congenital coloboma resulting from failure of
closure of the optic fissure include:

   1. coloboma of the choroid  3. coloboma of the iris
   2. coloboma of the retina   4. palpebral coloboma  A B C D E

| A | B | C | D | E |
|---|---|---|---|---|
| 1,2,3 | 1,3 | 2,4 | only 4 | all correct |

10. Structures derived from the branchial apparatus include:

   1. ear ossicles
   2. tympanic membrane

   3. auditory tube
   4. external acoustic meatus         A B C D E

======================= ANSWERS, NOTES, AND EXPLANATIONS =======================

1. A  1, 2, and 3 are correct.  The eyes develop from two germ layers:  ectoderm
   and mesoderm.  The retina differentiates from neuroectoderm and the lens is
   derived from surface ectoderm. The mesoderm gives rise to the extrinsic eye
   muscles and to connective and vascular tissues of the eyes.

2. C  2 and 4 are correct.  The three middle ear bones or ossicles develop on
   each side by endochondral ossification of the dorsal ends of the first arch
   cartilage or Meckel's cartilage (malleus and incus) and of the second arch
   cartilage or Reichert's cartilage (stapes).  These cartilages form the cartilaginous viscerocranium of the embryo.

3. E  All are correct.  The auditory system develops from all three germ layers.
   The otic vesicle or otocyst, which gives rise to the inner ear or membranous
   labyrinth, is derived from the surface ectoderm.  The epithelium lining the
   tympanic cavity, tympanic antrum, and auditory tube differentiates from the
   endodermal tubotympanic recess, a derivative of the first pharyngeal pouch.
   The epithelium of the external acoustic meatus is derived from the ectoderm
   of the first branchial groove.  The mesoderm gives rise to all muscles,
   connective tissue, cartilage, and bone in the ears.

4. C  2 and 4 are correct.  The retina and optic nerve develop from the optic
   vesicle which develops as an outgrowth of the brain.  The inner layer of the
   optic cup (invaginated optic vesicle) differentiates into the neural layer of
   the retina, and the outer layer becomes the pigmented epithelium.  The
   ventral (anterior) part of the optic cup forms the epithelium of the ciliary
   body and iris, as well as the iris muscles (sphincter and dilator of the
   pupil).  The fibers of the dilator, called myoepithelial cells, are not
   typical smooth muscle fibers.

5. B  1 and 3 are correct.  The cochlear duct develops from the ventral part of
   the otic vesicle, a derivative of the surface ectoderm.  This duct grows and
   coils to form the cochlea.  The corneal epithelium is the only part of the
   cornea derived from the surface ectoderm.  All other parts of it are derived
   from mesenchyme.  The highly vascularized pigment layer of the eye, known as
   the choroid posteriorly, develops from mesenchyme surrounding the developing
   eye.  The choroid is comparable to the pia mater of the brain.  The modiolus
   is the bony pillar or core around which the cochlea makes two and a half
   turns.  Like other bones, it is a mesodermal derivative.

6. D  Only 4 is correct.  The spiral organ (of Corti), the specialized organ of

hearing, is derived from the ventral portion of the otic vesicle. This complex receptor of auditory stimuli differentiates from the wall of the cochlear duct. The basilar membrane, composed of collagen fibers and sparse elastic fibers embedded in a ground substance, is derived from mesenchyme adjacent to the basilar region of the cochlear duct. The auricle (pinna) and the tympanic membrane are derivatives of the branchial apparatus.

7.  E  All are correct. Congenital cataracts are not uncommon. They may be unilateral or bilateral, but they are usually bilateral. Some cataracts are genetically determined, usually by dominant transmission. Other cataracts are caused by environmental factors. Though anoxia appears to play a part in some cases, and toxic causes have been suggested, maternal infections are the only well established environmental causes of congenital cataract. The risk of cataracts if maternal rubella infection occurs during the first four to six weeks, is as high as 50 percent. Often early infections result in a combination of cataract and heart defect. Cataracts also occur in toxoplasmosis and congenital syphilis. As these cataracts result from severe ocular inflammation during the later stages of pregnancy, they are often classified as secondary congenital cataracts.

8.  D  Only 4 is correct. In congenital glaucoma or buphthalmos, the intraocular pressure is above normal, and if not alleviated, will cause irreversible damage to the eye. The embryological basis of congenital glaucoma is an abnormal persistence of mesenchymal tissue in the angle of the anterior chamber of the eye. Usually this tissue disappears during the later fetal period and permits drainage of aqueous humor through the canal of Schlemm. Most cases of glaucoma are genetically determined; others are a complication of maternal rubella infection. As a result of the inadequate drainage of aqueous humor, the intraocular tension rises and the eye gradually enlarges.

9.  A  1, 2, and 3 are correct. Palpebral coloboma or a notch in the eyelid is rare and may be associated with coloboma iridis, but palpebral coloboma defects appear to result from a local developmental failure or disturbance in the margin of the optic cup. The other types of coloboma (1, 2, and 3) result from failure of the optic fissure on the inferior (caudal) surface of the optic cup to close during the sixth week. This leaves a cleft or coloboma in the eye. The defect is often partial, involving the choroid and retina, but it may extend anteriorly to involve the iris and ciliary body. Genetic factors, maternal infections (including rubella, toxoplasmosis) and radiation have been implicated as causes of optic fissure defects.

10. E  All are correct. The auditory ossicles are derived from the cartilages of the first two pairs of branchial arches. The tympanic membrane is the adult derivative of the first branchial membrane. The auditory tube is derived from the tubotympanic recess of the first pharyngeal pouch. The external acoustic meatus is the adult derivative of the first branchial groove.

F I V E - C H O I C E   A S S O C I A T I O N   Q U E S T I O N S

DIRECTIONS: Each group of questions below consists of a numbered list of descriptive words or phrases accompanied by a diagram with certain parts indicated by letters, or by a list of lettered headings. For each numbered word or phrase, SELECT THE LETTERED PART OR HEADING that matches it correctly. Then insert the letter in the space to the right of the appropriate number. Sometimes more than one numbered word or phrase may be correctly matched to the same lettered part or heading.

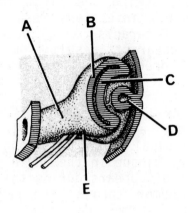

A. Sinus venosus sclerae
B. Optic nerve
C. Corneal epithelium
D. Central artery of retina
E. Pupillary membrane

1. _____ Becomes pigmented layer of the retina
2. _____ Optic fissure
3. _____ Becomes specialized for sensitivity to light
4. _____ Gives rise to the lens
5. _____ Future optic nerve
6. _____ Differentiates into nonpigmented portion of the ciliary epithelium

7. _____ Tunica vasculosa lentis
8. _____ Ganglion cells of the retina
9. _____ Hyaloid artery
10. _____ Surface ectoderm
11. _____ Congenital glaucoma
12. _____ Neuroectoderm

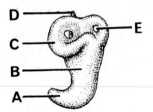

13. _____ Gives rise to a semicircular duct
14. _____ Absorption focus
15. _____ Endolymphatic duct
16. _____ Primordium of the cochlea
17. _____ Saccular portion of the otic vesicle
18. _____ Gives rise to the spiral organ

214

ASSOCIATION QUESTIONS

A. Conjunctival epithelium
B. Neuroectoderm
C. First pharyngeal pouch
D. First branchial groove
E. Mesenchyme

19. ____ External acoustic meatus
20. ____ Sclera and choroid
21. ____ Has same origin as cornea
22. ____ Mastoid cells
23. ____ Bipolar cells of the retina
24. ____ Tympanic cavity

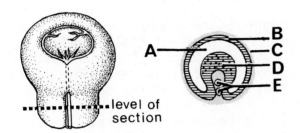

level of section

25. ____ Continuous with the pigmented epithelium of the retina
26. ____ Gradually obliterates
27. ____ Continuous with the neural layer of the retina
28. ____ Hyaloid vessels
29. ____ Continuous with the meninges
30. ____ Contains axons of ganglion cells

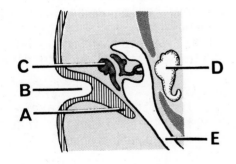

31. ____ Derived from Meckel's cartilage
32. ____ Gives rise to the utricle
33. ____ External acoustic meatus
34. ____ Meatal plug
35. ____ Derived from the tubotympanic recess
36. ____ Membranous labyrinth

========================= ANSWERS, NOTES, AND EXPLANATIONS =========================

1.  B  The outer layer of the optic cup differentiates into the pigmented layer of the retina.  The pigmented epithelium consists of a single layer of cells

that reinforces the light-absorbing properties of the choroid membrane to reduce scattering of light within the eye.

2. E  The optic fissure (choroidal or fetal fissure) develops on the inferior (caudal) surface of the optic cup and along the optic stalk. The hyaloid blood vessels pass into the optic cup along this groove and supply the lens and the developing neural layer of the retina.

3. C  The inner layer of the optic cup becomes the pars optica retinae or the neural layer of the retina. It differentiates into the visual receptive portion of the adult retina. The inner layer of the optic cup also gives rise to the pars ciliaris retinae and the pars iridis retinae.

4. D  The lens develops from the lens vesicle, a derivative of the surface ectoderm. The anterior wall of this vesicle becomes the anterior epithelium of the adult lens. Cells of the posterior wall lengthen to form lens fibers which grow into and gradually obliterate the cavity of the lens vesicle.

5. A  The optic stalk, connecting the optic cup to the brain, becomes the optic nerve as axons of ganglion cells in the neural layer of the retina pass into the inner wall of the stalk. As a result of the continually increasing number of optic nerve fibers, the inner wall of the stalk increases in thickness and fuses with the outer wall, obliterating the lumen of the optic stalk.

6. C  Most of the inner layer of the optic cup becomes the neural layer of the retina. The anterior part becomes the non-pigmented portion of the ciliary epithelium (ciliary portion of the retina) and the iridial portion of the retina. Toward the root of the iris, on the anterior surface of the ciliary processes, the cells of the inner layer of the cup gradually accumulate pigment granules.

7. E  The anterior portion of the tunica vasculosa lentis, a vascular layer around the embryonic lens, is called the pupillary membrane. When the distal portion of the hyaloid artery degenerates, the tunica vasculosa lentis, including the pupillary membrane, also degenerates. Remnants of this membrane often appear as tissue strands in normal eyes of infants, but these strands usually cause little disturbance of vision and they tend to disappear in old age.

8. B  As the neural layer of the retina develops from the inner layer of the optic cup, the axons of ganglion cells in the retina pass into the inner wall of the optic stalk and gradually convert it into the optic nerve.

9. D  The hyaloid artery passes via the optic fissure to the optic cup, where it supplies blood to the developing neural layer of the retina and to the embryonic lens. The distal portion of this artery usually degenerates, but the proximal portion persists as the central artery of the retina. Persistence of the distal portion of the hyaloid artery is a fairly common abnormality. It may persist in whole or in part, but it is usually not patent. The hyaloid arterial remnant appears as a thin line or thick cord in the vitreous humor (body).

10.  C  The corneal epithelium is derived from the surface ectoderm.  The lens functions as an inductor and influences the surface ectoderm to develop into the epithelium of the cornea.  The substantia propria of the cornea is derived from mesenchyme.

11.  A  Absence or incomplete development of the sinus venosus sclerae (canal of Schlemm) results in congenital glaucoma or buphthalmos.  This abnormality is usually caused by recessive mutant genes, but it sometimes results from a maternal rubella infection during early pregnancy.  The embryological basis of blockage or incomplete development of the canal of Schlemm is abnormal persistence of mesenchymal tissue in the angle of the anterior chamber.  As a result of inadequate drainage of the aqueous humor through the canal, intraocular tension rises and the eye gradually enlarges and the cornea becomes hazy.  Retinal damage causes visual impairment.

12.  B  The optic vesicle is an outgrowth of the brain.  Hence the retina and the optic nerve are derived from neuroectoderm of the embryonic brain.  The adult structure of the retina and optic nerve shows marked resemblance to the brain, and the coats of the eyeball and the optic nerve show resemblances to the coverings of the brain.  The central artery and vein of the retina pass in the meningeal sheaths and are included in the anterior part of the optic nerve.  This relationship is of clinical significance because an increase in pressure of cerebrospinal fluid around the optic nerve interferes with venous return from the eye, and edema of the optic disk (papilledema) results.  This is an important indicator of an increase in intracranial pressure.

13.  C  This flat disc-like diverticulum of the dorsal or utricular portion of the otic vesicle is the primordium of one of the three semicircular ducts.  They are attached to the utricle and later are enclosed in the semicircular canals of the bony labyrinth.  The sensory areas (cristae ampullares), which develop in these ducts, respond to changes in the direction of movement of the head.

14.  E  The central portions of the walls of the disc-like diverticula from the utricular portion of the otocyst fuse and later disappear.  Degeneration of tissue proceeds peripherally from the absorption focus, but peripheral portions of the diverticula remain as the semicircular ducts.  As the bony labyrinth forms around the ducts, they come to lie in semicircular canals.

15.  D  The endolymphatic duct appears as a hollow diverticulum from the dorsal utricular portion of the otocyst.  Its distal end expands to form the endolymphatic sac.

16.  A  The cochlear duct develops as a tubular diverticulum from the saccular portion of the otocyst.  The cochlear duct grows and makes two and a half turns around the developing modiolus, a bony pillar or core containing nerves and vessels.  The coiled cochlear duct is called the membranous cochlea and it is contained in the bony cochlea which develops from the surrounding mesenchyme.

17.  B  The saccular portion of the otic vesicle, called the saccule, is an

endolymph-containing dilation of the membranous labyrinth. The saccule contains a specialized area of sensory epithelium, the macula sacculi, and together with the macula utriculi, signals the orientation of the head in space.

18. A  The spiral organ (of Corti) differentiates from cells in the wall of the cochlear duct. Ganglion cells of the eighth cranial nerve migrate along the coils of the cochlea and form the cochlear (spiral) ganglion. Nerve processes grow from this ganglion to the spiral organ.

19. D  The external acoustic meatus is the adult derivative of the dorsal part of the first branchial groove. It grows inward as a funnel-shaped tube until it reaches the endodermal tubotympanic recess, the primordium of the tympanic cavity, tympanic antrum, auditory tube, and mastoid cells.

20. E  The sclera and choroid develop from mesenchyme surrounding the optic cup. The mesenchyme differentiates into an inner vascular layer, the choroid, and an outer fibrous layer, the sclera. Toward the margin of the optic cup, the choroid becomes modified to form the cores of the ciliary processes which consist chiefly of capillaries supported by delicate connective tissue.

21. A  The conjunctival epithelium, like the corneal epithelium, is derived from the surface ectoderm. The substantia (lamina) propria of the conjunctiva and of the cornea consists of connective tissue derived from mesenchyme. The conjunctiva is a thin transparent mucous membrane that covers the sclera of the eye and lines the eyelid. At the lid margin the epithelium of the conjunctiva becomes continuous with the epidermis of the skin, another derivative of the surface ectoderm.

22. C  The mastoid cells begin to develop near term as the endodermal lining of the tympanic cavity, a derivative of the first pharyngeal pouch, induces erosion of the bone around the ear. The epithelium lining the mastoid cells, formed by this process called pneumatization, is derived from endoderm. Most mastoid cells develop after birth.

23. B  The bipolar cells of the neural portion of the retina are derived from neuroectoderm of the brain. These cells are true neurons interposed between photoreceptor cells and ganglion cells.

24. C  The tympanic cavity develops from the expanded distal end of the tubotympanic recess, a derivative of the first pharyngeal pouch. The tympanic cavity is a tiny epithelium-lined cavity in bone that communicates with the nasopharynx through the auditory tube, another derivative of the first pharyngeal pouch.

25. B  The outer wall of the optic stalk is continuous with the outer wall of the optic cup which gives rise to the pigmented epithelium of the retina.

26. A  The lumen of the optic stalk gradually obliterates as the optic nerve forms. As the number of axons of ganglion cells from the retina increases in

the inner wall of the optic stalk, the lumen gradually disappears and the optic nerve forms.

27.   D  The inner layer of the optic stalk is continuous with the inner layer of the optic cup which gives rise to the neural layer of the retina.  The inner layer of the optic stalk thickens as axons of ganglion cells pass through it on their way to the brain.

28.   E  The hyaloid vessels supply blood to and return blood from the inner layer of the optic cup (future neural layer of retina) and the embryonic lens.  The distal portions of these vessels usually degenerate and the remaining parts become the central artery and vein of the retina.  When the optic fissure closes, these vessels are incorporated into the optic nerve.

29.   C  The sheath of the optic nerve is continuous with the meninges of the brain and with the choroid and sclera of the eye.  When the optic vesicles develop as outgrowths of the brain, they carry the layers of the meninges with them.

30.   D  The inner layer of the optic stalk contains axons of ganglion cells in the neural layer of the retina.  Eventually about one million fibers pass through the optic nerve, the adult derivative of the optic stalk.  The optic nerve fibers are myelinated by oligodendrocytes instead of by Schwann cells because the optic nerve is comparable to a tract within the brain.  The neuroepithelial cells in the walls of the optic stalk differentiate into oligodendrocytes and other neuroglial cells.

31.   C  The malleus, one of the middle ear bones or auditory ossicles, is derived from the first branchial arch cartilage or Meckel's cartilage.  It develops by endochondral ossification of the dorsal end of the cartilage.  The incus and stapes, the other two ossicles, are derived in a similar manner from the first and second branchial arch cartilages, respectively.

32.   D  The dorsal or utricular portion of the otic vesicle (otocyst) gives rise to the utricle.  Like the saccule, it is a dilation of the membranous labyrinth containing a specialized area of sensory epithelium, the macula utriculi.  The utricle and saccule are sensors of head movements.

33.   B  The external acoustic meatus is the adult derivative of the dorsal end of the first branchial groove.  This canal leads to the tympanic membrane and its function (along with the auricle) is to collect sound waves which cause resonant vibration of the tympanic membrane.

34.   A  The ectodermal cells at the bottom of the developing external acoustic meatus proliferate and grow caudally as a solid epithelial plate, called the meatal plug.  Late in fetal life, the central cells of this plug degenerate, forming the inner portion of the external acoustic meatus.  Failure of the meatal plug to canalize results in atresia of the external acoustic meatus and deafness.  This condition is usually caused by genetic factors.

35.   E  The auditory tube is derived from the tubotympanic recess, the embryonic derivative of the first pharyngeal pouch.  This tube makes possible adjustments of pressure in the middle ear.  When the tube opens during

219

swallowing, the pressure in the middle ear becomes equalized with the atmospheric pressure.

36.  D  The membranous labyrinth develops from the otic vesicle, a derivative of the surface ectoderm.  It gives rise to the utricle, saccule, endolymphatic duct and sac, semicircular ducts, and cochlea.  The internal ear, which has a dual function (hearing and equilibrium), consists of the membranous labyrinth derived from the otic vesicle.  It is enclosed in the bony labyrinth derived from the surrounding mesenchyme.

---

NOTES:

# THE INTEGUMENTARY SYSTEM

The Skin and Related Structures

## O B J E C T I V E S

BE ABLE TO:

---

o   Construct and label diagrams illustrating the development of skin, hair, nails, and sebaceous, sweat, and mammary glands.

o   Write explanatory notes on each of the following congenital malformations: ichthyosis, ectodermal dysplasia, athelia, amastia, polymastia, and polythelia.

o   Discuss the development of teeth using labeled sketches to illustrate the various stages of development.

o   Define the following terms: dental lamina, dental papilla, dental sac, epithelial root sheath, odontoblastic layer, odontoblastic processes, ameloblasts, and cementoblasts.

o   Describe eruption of the deciduous and permanent teeth.

o   Discuss the various causes of disturbances in enamel formation that result in enamel hypoplasia.

---

## F I V E - C H O I C E   C O M P L E T I O N   Q U E S T I O N S

DIRECTIONS: Each of the following statements or questions is followed by five suggested responses or completions. SELECT THE ONE BEST ANSWER in each case and then circle the appropriate letter at the right of each question.

1.  Each of the following structures is derived from the surface ectoderm except the

    A.  dental papilla            D.  sweat glands
    B.  fingernails               E.  tooth buds
    C.  epidermis
                                                          A B C D E

SELECT THE ONE BEST ANSWER

2. Which structure is <u>not</u> derived from the mesenchyme?

    A. Dental sac
    B. Dermal root sheath
    C. Arrector pili muscle
    D. Odontoblastic layer
    E. Epithelial root sheath                A B C D E

3. Which cells are derived from the neuroectoderm?

    A. Ameloblast           D. Melanoblast
    B. Odontoblast         E. Myoblast
    C. Cementoblast                    A B C D E

4. Most sebaceous glands develop as

    A. downgrowths of the stratum germinativum
    B. thickened areas of the epidermis
    C. buds from the sides of hair follicles
    D. downgrowths from the surface ectoderm
    E. ingrowths along the glandular ridges     A B C D E

5. The ameloblasts of the developing tooth produce

    A. predentin            D. periodontium
    B. dentin              E. enamel
    C. cementum                   A B C D E

6. The odontoblasts of the developing tooth produce

    A. predentin            D. periodontium
    B. dentin              E. enamel
    C. cementum                   A B C D E

7. Which of the following congenital malformations is common?

    A. Hypertrichosis
    B. Anonychia
    C. Ectodermal dysplasia
    D. Polymastia
    E. Anodontia                    A B C D E

8. Most congenital malformations of teeth are caused by

    A. tetracyclines        D. irradiation
    B. genetic factors      E. syphilis
    C. rubella virus                  A B C D E

======================= ANSWERS, NOTES, AND EXPLANATIONS =========================

1.  A   The dental papilla is a mass of condensed mesenchyme that invaginates the deep surface of the tooth bud.  The dental papilla gives rise to the dentin and the dental pulp.

2.  E   The epithelial root sheath of the hair follicle and of the developing tooth is derived from the surface ectoderm.  The dermal sheath (connective tissue) of the hair follicle, like the dental sac, is derived from mesenchyme.

3.  D   Melanoblasts are derived from the neural crest, a derivative of the neuroectoderm.  When the neural folds fuse to form the neural plate, some cells are not incorporated into it.  These cells form a neural crest which gives rise to the cells in the cranial, spinal, and autonomic ganglia, Schwann cells, melanoblasts, and cells of the suprarenal (adrenal) medulla.  If you chose B, you could be right because there is evidence suggesting that the odontoblasts differentiate from mesenchyme which is of neural crest origin.  However, D is the best answer because it is well established that melanoblasts are of neural crest origin.

4.  C   All sebaceous glands develop as buds from the sides of the developing epithelial root sheaths of hair follicles, except those in the glans penis, eyelids, nostrils, anal region, and labia minora.  In these sites, sebaceous glands develop as buds from the epidermis.

5.  E   The ameloblasts differentiate from the cells in the inner enamel epithelium of the enamel organ.  They produce enamel in the form of prisms (rods) and deposit it over the dentin.  Each melanoblast produces one enamel rod, the structural unit of enamel.  The ameloblasts degenerate after they have formed all the enamel and the tooth erupts.  Thus enamel is incapable of repair if it is injured by decay or injury.

6.  A   The odontoblasts produce predentin and deposit it adjacent to the inner enamel epithelium.  Later the predentin calcifies and becomes dentin.  Hence A is a better answer than B.

7.  D   An extra breast or mammary gland, called polymastia, is quite common.  About one percent of women have an extra breast or nipple.  These usually develop just inferior to the normal breast, but they may appear anywhere along the line of the embryonic mammary ridges that run from the axillae to the inguinal regions.

8.  B   Most congenital malformations of the teeth are hereditary in nature, i.e., they are caused by genetic factors.  The importance of genetic factors in tooth development and dental abnormalities is clearly demonstrated by studying the dentition in monozygotic twins.  Tetracycline, an antibiotic, crosses the placenta and is believed to cause minor tooth defects (enamel hypoplasia) and discoloration of the deciduous teeth.  Rubella virus, Treponema pallidum (the syphilis organism), and irradiation may also give rise to abnormalities of the teeth.  Nutritional deficiency, diseases such as measles, and high levels of fluoride may damage the ameloblasts and cause

defective enamel formation (enamel hypoplasia). Rickets resulting from a deficiency of vitamin D is, however, the most common cause of enamel hypoplasia. Abnormally shaped teeth are relatively common. Occasionally aberrant groups of ameloblasts give rise to spherical masses of enamel, called enamel pearls (drops), which often project from the side of the tooth.

## M U L T I - C O M P L E T I O N   Q U E S T I O N S

DIRECTIONS: In each of the following questions or incomplete statements ONE OR MORE of the completions is correct. At the lower right of each question, circle A if 1, 2, and 3 are correct; B if 1 and 3 are correct; C if 2 and 4 are correct; D if only 4 is correct; and E if all are correct.

1. Parts of a developing hair, derived from the epidermis include:

   1. germinal matrix
   2. epithelial root sheath
   3. hair bulb
   4. dermal hair sheath            A B C D E

2. Cells derived from the oral ectoderm include:

   1. cementoblasts
   2. melanoblasts
   3. odontoblasts
   4. ameloblasts                   A B C D E

3. Sebaceous glands develop from the surface ectoderm in which of the following sites:

   1. palms of the hand
   2. labia minora
   3. soles of the feet
   4. eyelids                       A B C D E

4. During development of the tooth, mesenchymal cells give rise to the

   1. periodontal ligament
   2. odontoblastic layer
   3. dental sac
   4. root sheath                   A B C D E

5. Sweat glands develop from the surface ectoderm in which of the following sites:

   1. palms of the hand
   2. labia majora
   3. soles of the feet
   4. margins of the lips           A B C D E

6. The dental laminae give rise to the

   1. tooth buds for the deciduous teeth
   2. enamel organs of the developing teeth
   3. tooth buds for the permanent teeth
   4. enamel reticulum of the developing teeth    A B C D E

| A | B | C | D | E |
|---|---|---|---|---|
| 1,2,3 | 1,3 | 2,4 | only 4 | all correct |

7. The mesenchyme in the dental papilla gives rise to the

    1. dental follicle
    2. dental pulp
    3. dental sac
    4. dentin                                A B C D E

8. Common congenital malformations of the mammary glands include:

    1. polymastia
    2. amastia
    3. polythelia
    4. athelia                               A B C D E

9. Supernumerary breasts or nipples may appear in which of the following sites?

    1. Medial side of thighs
    2. Anterior abdominal wall
    3. Inguinal region
    4. Axillary region                     A B C D E

10. Tetracycline antibiotics may produce brownish-yellow discoloration of the teeth and enamel hypoplasia if administered during which of the following periods?

    1. infancy
    2. fetal period
    3. childhood
    4. embryonic period                  A B C D E

======================= ANSWERS, NOTES, AND EXPLANATIONS =======================

1. A **1, 2, and 3 are correct.** Hairs develop as solid cylindrical downgrowths of the epidermis into the underlying mesenchyme. The tip of each downgrowth, the hair bulb, grows around a vascular mesenchymal condensation, the hair papilla. The peripheral cells of the epidermal downgrowth form the inner or epithelial root sheath, and the surrounding mesenchymal cells condense to form the outer or dermal root sheath.

2. D **4 only is correct.** The ameloblasts are derived from the inner enamel epithelium of the enamel organ which is derived from the oral ectoderm (in-

vaginated surface ectoderm). The melanoblasts are derived from the neural crest, a derivative of the neuroectoderm.

3.  C  2 and 4 are correct.  Most sebaceous glands develop as outgrowths from hair follicles, explaining why there are none of these glands in the palms of the hands and the soles of the feet.  However, sebaceous glands develop without hair follicles in a few sites, e.g., in the lips, eyelids, papillae of breasts, labia minora, and glans penis.

4.  A  1, 2, and 3 are correct.  The dental sac is derived from the mesenchyme surrounding the developing tooth.  The periodontal ligament, a derivative of the dental sac, holds the tooth in its bony socket or alveolus.  The odontoblastic layer develops from the mesenchymal cells adjacent to the inner enamel epithelium of the enamel organ.  The epithelial root sheath develops from the inner and outer epithelia where they come together in the neck region of the tooth.  The enamel epithelia are derived from the oral ectoderm.

5.  A  1, 2, and 3 are correct.  Ordinary sweat glands (i.e., the eccrine type) develop as downgrowths of the epidermis.  No sweat glands develop in the red margins of the lips.  The apocrine sweat glands (e.g., in the axilla) develop as outgrowths of the hair follicles in a manner similar to the development of most sebaceous glands.

6.  E  All are correct.  The dental laminae are U-shaped thickenings of the oral epithelium (ectoderm) which give rise to the buds for the deciduous and permanent teeth.  The enamel organs develop as the tooth buds are invaginated by mesenchyme, called the dental papilla.  The enamel (stellate) reticulum is the core of loosely arranged cells located between the inner and outer layers of enamel epithelium of the enamel organ.

7.  C  2 and 4 are correct.  The dental papilla is a mass of condensed mesenchyme that invaginates the tooth bud, converting it into a cap-shaped structure. The dental papilla later becomes the pulp of the tooth.  The mesenchymal cells in the dental papilla adjacent to the inner enamel epithelium differentiate into odontoblasts.  These cells produce predentin which later calcifies to form dentin.  The dental sac or follicle is a capsule-like structure that develops around the developing tooth from the surrounding mesenchyme.  The cementoblasts of the dental sac (dental follicle) produce cementum.  This sac also gives rise to the periodontal ligament which holds the tooth in its socket.

8.  B  1 and 3 are correct.  An extra breast (polymastia) or nipple (polythelia) occurs in about one percent of women.  Both are inheritable conditions.  The extra breast or nipple usually develops just below the normal breast or in the axilla.

9.  E  All are correct.  Mammary glands develop as solid downgrowths of the epidermis along the embryonic mammary ridges which extend from the axillary region to the inguinal region.  Usually mammary glands develop only in the thoracic (pectoral) region, but they may develop anywhere from the axilla to the thigh regions, along the lines of the embryonic mammary ridges.  An extra

breast usually appears just inferior to the normal one.

10. A  1, 2, and 3 are correct.  Foreign substances are sometimes incorporated into developing enamel and they may affect enamel development if administered during the period of enamel formation.  This period extends from about 20 fetal weeks until about 16 years.  The enamel is completely formed on all but the third molars by the eighth year.  If possible, therefore, tetracyclines should not be prescribed for pregnant women or for children under eight years of age because of the possibility of producing discoloration of the deciduous and/or permanent teeth.  Discoloration of teeth has been observed following administration of all the tetracycline antibiotics.

## F I V E - C H O I C E   A S S O C I A T I O N   Q U E S T I O N S

DIRECTIONS:  Each group of questions below consists of a numbered list of descriptive words or phrases accompanied by a diagram with certain parts indicated by letters, or by a list of lettered headings.  For each numbered word or phrase, SELECT THE LETTERED PART OR HEADING that matches it correctly.  Then insert the letter in the space to the right of the appropriate number.  Sometimes more than one numbered word or phrase may be correctly matched to the same lettered part or heading.

A. Dental pulp
B. Predentin
C. Dental sac
D. Enamel
E. Cementum

1. ____ Periodontal ligament
2. ____ Odontoblasts
3. ____ Inner enamel epithelium
4. ____ Contains vessels and nerves
5. ____ Ameloblasts
6. ____ Inner cells of dental sac

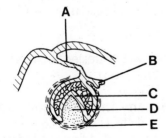

7. ____ Inner enamel epithelium
8. ____ Dental sac
9. ____ Dental lamina
10. ____ Dental papilla
11. ____ Bud of permanent tooth
12. ____ Part of the enamel organ

## ASSOCIATION QUESTIONS

A. Tetracyclines
B. Ameloblastic layer
C. Hair follicles
D. Neural crest cells
E. Epithelial root sheath
   of the developing tooth

13. ____ Melanocytes
14. ____ Induction of odontoblastic layer
15. ____ Lanugo
16. ____ Discoloration of the teeth
17. ____ Sebaceous glands
18. ____ Fused layers of enamel epithelia
19. ____ Derived from the inner enamel epithelium
20. ____ Derived from the neural plate

======================= ANSWERS, NOTES, AND EXPLANATIONS =========================

1. C  The periodontal ligament is derived from the dental sac, a capsule-like structure that develops from the mesenchyme surrounding the tooth.

2. B  The odontoblasts derived from mesenchymal cells in the dental papilla (future pulp) give rise to predentin and deposit it adjacent to the inner enamel epithelium. Later the predentin calcifies and becomes dentin.

3. D  Cells of the inner enamel epithelium adjacent to the dentin differentiate into ameloblasts. These cells produce enamel in the form of prisms (rods) and deposit over the dentin.

4. A  The dental pulp derived from the mesenchymal dental papilla of the embryo contains the vessels and nerves of the tooth.

5. D  The ameloblasts are enamel formers. They produce long enamel prisms and deposit them over the dentin. Enamel formation begins at about 20 weeks in the deciduous teeth and continues in the permanent teeth until about 16 years of age. If vitamin D is deficient during this period, the erupted surfaces of the teeth may be rough instead of smooth and shiny. The ameloblastic layer also induces the odontoblastic layer to form. Hence, if the ameloblasts do not differentiate normally (e.g., as in vitamin A deficiency), dentin formation is also affected.

6. E  The inner cells of the dental sac differentiate into cementoblasts which produce cementum and deposit it over the dentin of the root.

7. C  The inner enamel epithelium of the enamel organ induces the adjacent mesenchymal cells in the dental papilla to differentiate into an odontoblastic layer. The inner enamel epithelium differentiates into ameloblasts, the enamel-forming cells.

8.  E  The dental sac develops from the mesenchyme surrounding the developing tooth. This capsule-like structure gives rise to cementoblasts which form cementum, and to the periodontal ligament which embeds in the cementum and the surrounding bony socket of the tooth. Thus, the periodontal ligament holds the tooth in its socket.

9.  A  The dental lamina develops from the oral ectoderm and gives rise to the deciduous and permanent tooth buds.

10. D  The dental papilla, a condensation of mesenchyme, invaginates the tooth bud, giving it the appearance of a cap. The dental papilla gives rise to the dental pulp and to the odontoblasts which form the dentin. There is some evidence that the mesenchymal cells that differentiate into odontoblasts are derived from the neural crest.

11. B  The tooth buds for the permanent teeth develop from continuations of the dental laminae. They begin to appear at about 10 weeks and lie lingual to the deciduous tooth buds.

12. C  The inner enamel epithelium is part of the enamel organ. Other parts are the outer enamel epithelium and the enamel recticulum. For a while the enamel organ is attached to the oral epithelium by the dental lamina.

13. D  Melanocytes differentiate from melanoblasts which are derived from neural crest cells. Melanoblasts migrate into the dermis during the early fetal period and soon enter the epidermis where they differentiate into melanocytes. These cells produce melanin and distribute it to the epidermal cells after birth. Melanoblasts also migrate into the hair bulbs and differentiate into melanocytes. Melanin is distributed to the hair-forming cells before birth.

14. B  The ameloblastic layer induces the mesenchymal cells in the dental papilla adjacent to the inner enamel epithelium, to differentiate into odontoblasts. If there is a deficiency of vitamin A, the ameloblasts do not differentiate properly. Consequently, there is abnormal formation of odontoblasts.

15. C  Lanugo is the name given to the soft downy hairs that are first produced by the hair follicles. These hairs are chiefly shed before or right after birth and are replaced by coarser hairs which arise from new hair follicles.

16. A  Tetracycline antibiotics are known to cause brownish-yellow discoloration and fetal enamel hypoplasia if given to pregnant females or to children. If given after the eighth year, the third molar teeth are the only ones that may be affected because they are still developing.

17. C  Most sebaceous glands arise as buds from the sides of the epithelial root sheaths of hair follicles, late in the second trimester of pregnancy. A few sebaceous glands develop from the epidermis, independently of hair follicles (e.g., in the eyelids and labia minora).

18. E  The inner and outer enamel epithelia of the enamel organ come together and fuse in the neck region of the tooth, where they form the epithelial root

sheath.  This sheath grows into the mesenchyme and initiates root formation.

19.   B  The ameloblastic layer is derived from the inner enamel epithelium of the enamel organ.  The ameloblasts produce enamel and deposit it over the dentin. As the enamel increases, the ameloblasts regress toward the outer enamel epithelium.  Enamel and dentin formation begins at the tip (cusp) of the tooth and progresses toward the future root.

20.   D  The neural crest cells are derived from the neuroepithelium of the neural plate.  When the neural folds fuse, some neuroectodermal cells at the lateral edges of the neural plate are not incorporated into the neural tube; these cells form the neural crest that give rise to neural crest cells.

NOTES:

REVIEW EXAMINATION

INTRODUCTORY NOTE: The following 125 multiple-choice questions are based on all chapters in this Study Guide and Review Manual. You should be able to answer these questions in one and a half hours. The key to the correct responses is on page Number 247.

### F I V E - C H O I C E   C O M P L E T I O N   Q U E S T I O N S

DIRECTIONS: Each of the following statements or questions is followed by five suggested responses or completions. SELECT THE ONE BEST ANSWER in each case and then circle the appropriate letter at the right of each question.

1. Which statement about a 14-day blastocyst is _false_?

   A. Extraembryonic coelom surrounds the yolk sac.
   B. Chorionic villi are absent.
   C. A primitive uteroplacental circulation is established.
   D. The extraembryonic mesoderm is split into two layers.
   E. None of the above.                                     A B C D E

2. Morphologically abnormal sperms are generally believed to cause

   A. monosomy                    D. Klinefelter syndrome
   B. congenital abnormalities    E. none of the above
   C. trisomy                                                A B C D E

3. The notochordal process lengthens by addition of cells from the

   A. notochord                   D. primitive knot
   B. primitive streak            E. primitive groove
   C. notochordal plate                                      A B C D E

4. During the early part of the fourth week, the rate of growth at the periphery of the embryonic disc fails to keep pace with rate of growth of the

   A. yolk sac                    D. amniotic cavity
   B. neural tube                 E. primitive gut
   C. embryonic coelom                                       A B C D E

<u>SELECT THE ONE BEST ANSWER</u>

5. Derivatives of the first pharyngeal pouch include:

   A. tympanic antrum
   B. tubotympanic recess
   C. tympanic cavity
   D. auditory tube
   E. all of the above

   A B C D E

6. Known causes of microcephaly include each of the following <u>except</u>:

   A. rubella (German measles)
   B. cytomegalovirus
   C. thalidomide
   D. therapeutic radiation
   E. <u>Toxoplasma gondii</u>

   A B C D E

7. Each of the following would be good advice to give a woman who has just missed a menstrual period and may be pregnant, <u>except</u>:

   A. Obtain a vaccination against rubella infection.
   B. Avoid exposure to radiations whether for diagnostic or therapeutic purposes.
   C. Do not take any drugs that are not prescribed by a medical doctor.
   D. Stay away from persons with infectious diseases.
   E. Eat a good quality diet and do not smoke.

   A B C D E

8. An examination of the placenta and fetal membranes of male twins revealed two amnions, two chorions, and fused placentas. Twinning most likely resulted from

   A. dispermy
   B. fertilization of two ova
   C. superfecundation
   D. fertilization of one ovum
   E. treatment with gonadotropins

   A B C D E

9. Structures derived from the fourth pair of pharyngeal pouches include:

   A. Hassall's corpuscles
   B. thymus gland
   C. superior parathyroid glands
   D. inferior parathyroid glands
   E. all of the above

   A B C D E

10. The right auricle of the heart is derived from the

    A. primitive pulmonary vein
    B. sinus venosus
    C. right pulmonary vein
    D. sinus venarum
    E. primitive atrium

    A B C D E

## SELECT THE ONE BEST ANSWER

11. Each of the following structures is part of the first branchial arch except the

    A. facial nerve
    B. mandibular prominence
    C. Meckel's cartilage
    D. primordium of the malleus
    E. maxillary prominence

    A B C D E

12. In humans, cleft lip with or without cleft palate usually results from

    A. riboflavin deficiency
    B. infectious diseases
    C. irradiation
    D. cortisone
    E. mutant genes

    A B C D E

13. Which of the following is most likely to cause severe congenital malformations in human embryos?

    A. Cortisone
    B. Potassium iodide
    C. Aminopterin
    D. Lysergic acid
    E. Norethynodrel

    A B C D E

14. The most distinctive characteristic of a primary chorionic villus is its

    A. outer syncytial layer
    B. cytotrophoblastic core
    C. villous appearance
    D. mesenchymal core
    E. cytotrophoblastic shell

    A B C D E

15. A newborn infant with ambiguous genitalia was found to have chromatin negative nuclei. Gonads were palpable in the inguinal canals. The phallus was short and curved (chordee). There was no family history of intersexuality. What is the most likely diagnosis?

    A. perineal hypospadias
    B. gonadal dysgenesis
    C. male pseudohermaphroditism
    D. female pseudohermaphroditism
    E. true hermaphroditism

    A B C D E

16. Amniocentesis and amniotic fluid examination are most commonly used to

    A. diagnose chromosomal sex
    B. detect placental insufficiency
    C. determine the composition of the fluid
    D. detect chromosomal abnormalities
    E. diagnose a multiple gestation

    A B C D E

SELECT THE ONE BEST ANSWER

17. Narrowing of the lumen in pyloric stenosis usually results from

    A. hypertrophy of the longitudinal muscular layer
    B. a diaphragm-like narrowing of the pyloric lumen
    C. persistence of the solid stage of pyloric development
    D. hypertrophy of the circular muscular layer
    E. a so-called 'fetal vascular accident'                          A B C D E

18. Which of the following cells produce pulmonary surfactant?

    A. Type I alveolar epithelial cells
    B. Type II alveolar epithelial cells
    C. Alveolar macrophages (phagocytes)
    D. Pulmonary epithelial cells
    E. Endothelial cells                                              A B C D E

19. You examine a newborn infant and observe ambiguous external genitalia. Buccal smears show chromatin positive nuclei. Then you detect an elevated 17-ketosteroid output. What is the most likely diagnosis?

    A. Gonadal dysgenesis resulting from chromosomal abnormalities
    B. Female pseudohermaphroditism caused by maternal androgens
    C. Congenital virilizing adrenocortical hyperplasia
    D. Male infant with perineal hypospadias
    E. Familial male pseudohermaphroditism                           A B C D E

20. Anorectal agenesis is usually associated with a rectourethral fistula. The embryological basis of the fistula is

    A. abnormal partitioning of the cloaca
    B. agenesis of the urorectal septum
    C. failure of fixation of the hindgut
    D. failure of the proctodeum to develop
    E. premature rupture of the anal membrane                        A B C D E

21. Congenital heart disease most frequently results from

    A. maternal medications
    B. rubella virus
    C. mutant genes
    D. fetal distress
    E. genetic and environmental factors                             A B C D E

## SELECT THE ONE BEST ANSWER

22. The primordial germ cells are first observed in the

    A. dorsal mesentery
    B. primary sex cords
    C. gonadal ridges
    D. wall of the yolk sac
    E. mesoderm of the
       allantois

    A B C D E

23. As the metanephric diverticulum grows it becomes capped
    by ____ mesoderm.

    A. splanchnic
    B. mesonephric
    C. metanephric
    D. somatic
    E. intermediate

    A B C D E

24. The most common type of anorectal malformation is

    A. anal stenosis
    B. anorectal agenesis
    C. ectopic anus
    D. anal agenesis
    E. persistent anal
       membrane

    A B C D E

25. The most common cause of female pseudohermaphroditism is

    A. androgenic hormone ingestion
    B. adrenocortical hyperplasia
    C. arrhenoblastoma in the mother
    D. testicular feminization
    E. maternal progestins

    A B C D E

26. A fetus born prematurely during which of the following
    periods of lung development may survive?

    A. Organogenetic
    B. Canalicular
    C. Pseudoglandular
    D. Terminal sac
    E. Embryonic

    A B C D E

27. Exstrophy of the bladder is often associated with

    A. adrenocortical hyperplasia
    B. epispadias
    C. hypospadias
    D. urachal fistula
    E. chromosomal
       abnormalities

    A B C D E

28. The most common congenital malformation of the heart and
    great vessels associated with the congenital rubella
    syndrome is

    A. coarctation of the aorta
    B. tetralogy of Fallot
    C. patent ductus arteriosus
    D. atrial septal defect
    E. ventricular septal defect

    A B C D E

SELECT THE ONE BEST ANSWER

29. The mesonephric duct in male embryos gives rise to the

    A. ductus deferens          D. duct of epoophoron
    B. duct of Gartner          E. rete testis
    C. ductuli efferentes                                      A B C D E

30. Hematopoiesis begins during the ____ week of development.

    A. third                    D. sixth
    B. fourth                   E. seventh
    C. fifth                                                   A B C D E

31. The most common type of accessory rib is

    A. cervical                 D. thoracic
    B. sacral                   E. lumbar
    C. fused                                                   A B C D E

32. The ameloblasts of the developing tooth produce

    A. predentin                D. enamel
    B. dentin                   E. periodontium
    C. cementum                                                A B C D E

33. Which of the following structures is <u>not</u> derived from mesoderm?

    A. Choroid                  D. Sclera
    B. Membranous labyrinth     E. Bony labyrinth
    C. Extrinsic eye muscles                                   A B C D E

34. The myelin sheath of a peripheral nerve fiber is formed by

    A. mesenchymal cells        D. neural crest cells
    B. neuroepithelial cells    E. microglia
    C. Schwann cells                                           A B C D E

35. Teratogens acting after the ____ week will not cause limb malformations.

    A. fourth                   D. seventh
    B. fifth                    E. eighth
    C. sixth                                                   A B C D E

36. At birth the inferior end of the spinal cord usually lies at the level of the ____ vertebra.

    A. first sacral             D. third lumbar
    B. third sacral             E. twelfth thoracic
    C. first lumbar                                            A B C D E

<u>SELECT THE ONE BEST ANSWER</u>

37. Structures derived from ectoderm include:

    A. external acoustic meatus
    B. otic vesicle
    C. corneal epithelium
    D. lens
    E. all of the above                    A B C D E

38. Cellular components of the retina derived from the inner
    layer of the optic cup include:

    A. rod cells
    B. ganglion cells
    C. neuroglial cells
    D. bipolar cells
    E. all of the above                    A B C D E

39. The myelin sheaths surrounding axons in the central
    nervous system are formed by

    A. neuroglial cells
    B. astrocytes
    C. oligodendrocytes
    D. microglial cells
    E. Schwann cells                       A B C D E

40. Myoblasts from the occipital myotomes give rise to
    muscles of the

    A. neck          D. tongue
    B. ear           E. pharynx
    C. eye                                 A B C D E

41. Most congenital malformations of teeth are caused by

    A. rubella virus     D. irradiation
    B. genetic factors   E. syphilis
    C. tetracyclines                       A B C D E

42. Conditions known to follow infection with cytomegalo-
    virus or <u>Toxoplasma</u> <u>gondii</u> during the fetal period
    include:

    A. mental retardation
    B. hydrocephaly
    C. microcephaly
    D. microphthalmia
    E. all of the above                    A B C D E

# M U L T I - C O M P L E T I O N   Q U E S T I O N S

DIRECTIONS:   In each of the following questions or incomplete statements ONE OR MORE of the completions is correct.  At the lower right of each question, circle A if 1, 2, and 3 are correct;  B if 1 and 3  are correct;  C if 2 and 4 are correct;  D if only 4 is correct; and E if all are correct.


43.   Events occurring during the fourth week include:

1.  limb buds appear
2.  somites form
3.  neuropores close
4.  neural folds fuse

A B C D E

44.   True statements about the chorionic sac include:

1.  It contains the conceptus.
2.  Its walls consist of extraembryonic mesoderm and trophoblast.
3.  It rarely develops in ectopic pregnancies.
4.  The embryo is connected to its wall.

A B C D E

45.   The human morula

1.  consists of 16 or so blastomeres
2.  enters the uterus three days after conception
3.  forms about three days after fertilization
4.  contains a single fluid-filled cavity

A B C D E

46.   Before fertilizing an ovum, a sperm must

1.  undergo a physiological change called capacitation
2.  completely penetrate the corona radiata and the zona pellucida
3.  undergo a structural change called the acrosomal reaction
4.  complete the second meiotic division

A B C D E

47.   Structures involved in formation of the notochord include:

1.  primitive streak
2.  notochordal plate
3.  embryonic endoderm
4.  notochordal process

A B C D E

48.   Remnants of the primitive streak are most likely to

1.  appear in the sacrococcygeal region
2.  give rise to tumors in females
3.  give rise to a sacrococcygeal teratoma
4.  give rise to chordomas

A B C D E

| A | B | C | D | E |
|---|---|---|---|---|
| 1,2,3 | 1,3 | 2,4 | only 4 | all correct |

49. You detect a painless swelling in the midline of the neck in an infant just inferior to the hyoid bone. You observe that the mass moves superiorly when the tongue is protruded or during swallowing. From your embryological knowledge, what would you include in the differential diagnosis?

    1. Branchial cyst
    2. Thyroglossal duct cyst
    3. Branchial vestige
    4. Ectopic thyroid gland

    A B C D E

50. Abnormal transformation of first branchial arch components into their adult derivatives may give rise to which of the following congenital malformations?

    1. Hypoplasia of the mandible
    2. Cleft of the posterior palate
    3. Malformed external ear
    4. Fish-mouth deformity

    A B C D E

51. Unilateral cleft of the posterior palate results from failure of the lateral palatine process on the affected side to fuse with the

    1. median palatine process
    2. the other lateral palatine process
    3. mesenchyme in the primitive palate
    4. nasal septum

    A B C D E

52. Chromosome complements associated with recognizable congenital malformations in newborn infants include:

    1. 45,XO                    3. 47,XX
    2. 47,XXX                   4. 47,XXY

    A B C D E

53. Syndromes that do not usually exhibit severe mental retardation as a characteristic include:

    1. Down syndrome (trisomy 21)
    2. Klinefelter syndrome (47,XXY)
    3. Edwards syndrome (trisomy 18)
    4. Turner syndrome (45,XO)

    A B C D E

54. During tooth development mesenchymal cells give rise to the

    1. odontoblastic layer          3. dental sac
    2. periodontal ligament         4. root sheath

    A B C D E

| A | B | C | D | E |
|---|---|---|---|---|
| 1,2,3 | 1,3 | 2,4 | only 4 | all correct |

55. The kinds of information that routine sex chromatin tests provide concerning the sex chromosome complements include:

    1. anomalies of the Y-chromosome
    2. monosomy of a sex chromosome
    3. structural abnormalities
    4. the number of X-chromosomes

    A B C D E

56. A newborn infant was observed to have a low birth weight and bilateral congenital cataracts. Subsequently a patent ductus arteriosus was detected and the infant was found to be deaf. Probable causes of these abnormalities include:

    1. malnutrition and maternal smoking
    2. diagnostic x-rays during the first trimester
    3. toxoplasmosis during the second trimester
    4. German measles during the first trimester

    A B C D E

57. The placental membrane

    1. becomes relatively thinner as pregnancy advances
    2. is interposed between the fetal and maternal blood
    3. initially consists of four layers of embryonic tissue
    4. is composed entirely of tissues of fetal origin

    A B C D E

58. The embryological basis of thymic aplasia and absence of the parathyroid glands is failure of differentiation of the

    1. ventral portions of the third pair of pharyngeal pouches
    2. dorsal portions of the third pair of pharyngeal pouches
    3. dorsal portions of the fourth pair of pharyngeal pouches
    4. ventral portions of the fourth pair of pharyngeal pouches

    A B C D E

59. Correct statements concerning innervation of the developing diaphragm include:

    1. The phrenic nerves pass to the diaphragm via the pleuro-pericardial membranes.
    2. The sole motor nerve supply of the diaphragm is from the third, fourth, and fifth cervical segments of the spinal cord.
    3. Marginal branches are supplied to the diaphragm by the intercostal nerves.
    4. The phrenic nerves form during the fourth and fifth weeks as the diaphragm is developing.

    A B C D E

| A | B | C | D | E |
|---|---|---|---|---|
| 1,2,3 | 1,3 | 2,4 | only 4 | all correct |

60. Fetal growth is known to be affected adversely by.

    1. impaired uteroplacental blood flow
    2. severe maternal malnutrition
    3. placental insufficiency
    4. heavy cigarette smoking                          A B C D E

61. Correct statements about hypospadias include:

    1. It may produce ambiguous external genitalia.
    2. It is an uncommon condition in males.
    3. It is often associated with cryptorchidism.
    4. It is unrelated to intersexuality.                A B C D E

62. Findings consistent with a diagnosis of female pseudo-
    hermaphroditism due to congenital virilizing adrenal
    hyperplasia include:

    1. an enlarged clitoris
    2. fused labioscrotal folds
    3. an elevated 17-ketosteroid output
    4. chromatin-negative nuclei                         A B C D E

63. Hyaline membrane disease is

    1. commonly associated with polyhydramnios
    2. principally a disease of premature infants
    3. caused by overdistention of alveoli
    4. associated with a deficiency of surfactant        A B C D E

64. Tracheoesophageal fistula

    1. is commonly associated with esophageal atresia
    2. commonly joins the esophagus to the trachea near
       its bifurcation
    3. is encountered more often in males than in females
    4. results from unequal partitioning of the foregut into
       the esophagus and trachea                         A B C D E

65. Congenital inguinal hernia is

    1. often associated with cryptorchidism
    2. the result of a persistent processus vaginalis
    3. more common in males than in females
    4. usually of the direct type                        A B C D E

| A<br>1,2,3 | B<br>1,3 | C<br>2,4 | D<br>only 4 | E<br>all correct |
|---|---|---|---|---|

66. A newborn infant coughs and regurgitates its milk when fed, and has respiratory distress and abdominal distention when it cries. Congenital malformations that would most likely be considered in the differential diagnosis of the infant's problems include:

    1. agenesis of a lung
    2. tracheoesophageal fistula
    3. tracheal atresia
    4. esophageal atresia          A B C D E

67. Patent ductus arteriosus (PDA) is

    1. associated with rubella
    2. more frequent in females
    3. an aortic arch anomaly
    4. a common malformation      A B C D E

68. The permanent kidney is derived from the

    1. mesonephric tubules
    2. metanephric diverticulum
    3. paraxial mesoderm
    4. nephrogenic cord            A B C D E

69. Correct statements about intestinal atresia include:

    1. Atresias are most common in the ileum.
    2. Duodenal atresia may be associated with polyhydramnios.
    3. Atresias are associated with vomiting and abdominal distention.
    4. Atresia is less common than stenosis.          A B C D E

70. Exstrophy of the bladder (ectopia vesicae) is

    1. more common in males than in females
    2. caused by a failure of migration of mesenchymal cells
    3. accompanied by defective anterior abdominal muscles
    4. associated with epispadias          A B C D E

71. Embryological bases of chronic discharges from the umbilicus include:

    1. umbilico-ileal fistula
    2. umbilical sinus
    3. urachal sinus
    4. urachal fistula            A B C D E

72. A laboratory report states that chromatin-positive nuclei are present in the oral epithelial cells of a buccal smear. The smear could have been taken from a

    1. normal female
    2. female with the Down syndrome
    3. 47,XXY male

|  | A<br>1,2,3 | B<br>1,3 | C<br>2,4 | D<br>only 4 | E<br>all correct |
| --- | --- | --- | --- | --- | --- |

73. Doubling of the collecting system of the kidney results from

    1. incomplete division of the metanephric diverticulum
    2. persistence of vessels that normally disappear
    3. complete division of the metanephric diverticulum
    4. a deficiency of metanephric mesoderm          A B C D E

74. The auditory system is derived from the

    1. first branchial groove        3. mesoderm
    2. first pharyngeal pouch         4. endoderm          A B C D E

75. Malformations associated with spina bifida with meningo-
    myelocele include:

    1. Arnold-Chiari malformation    3. clubfoot
    2. vertebral arch defect         4. amyelia          A B C D E

76. Absence or incomplete development of the canal of Schlemm
    causes

    1. coloboma                      3. ectopia lentis
    2. megalocornea                  4. glaucoma          A B C D E

77. The Schwann cells give rise to the

    1. endoneurium                   3. perineurium
    2. myelin sheath                 4. neurolemma          A B C D E

78. Conditions often associated with spina bifida cystica
    include:

    1. hydrocephalus                 3. neurological deficit
    2. loss of sensation             4. muscle paralysis          A B C D E

79. Cells derived from the oral ectoderm include:

    1. cementoblasts                 3. melanoblasts
    2. odontoblasts                  4. ameloblasts          A B C D E

80. Structures derived from the neuroectoderm include:

    1. lens                          3. corneal epithelium
    2. iris muscles                  4. retina          A B C D E

81. Structures derived from the branchial apparatus include:

    1. auditory tube                 3. tympanic antrum
    2. external acoustic meatus      4. tympanic membrane          A B C D E

| A | B | C | D | E |
|---|---|---|---|---|
| 1,2,3 | 1,3 | 2,4 | only 4 | all correct |

82. Common causes of limb malformations <u>nowadays</u> include:

    1. mechanical factors
    2. thalidomide
    3. infectious agents
    4. genetic factors                    A B C D E

83. Tetracycline antibiotics may produce discoloration of the teeth and enamel hypoplasia if administered during

    1. infancy          3. fetal period
    2. childhood        4. embryonic period    A B C D E

84. The eyes are derived from

    1. surface ectoderm
    2. neuroectoderm
    3. mesoderm
    4. first pharyngeal pouch              A B C D E

85. Spina bifida cystica usually occurs in which of the following regions:

    1. coccygeal       3. cervical
    2. lumbar          4. sacral             A B C D E

86. Parts of the auditory system derived from the otic vesicle include:

    1. tympanic cavity    3. auricle
    2. tympanic membrane  4. spiral organ    A B C D E

87. Bones that form part of the neurocranium include:

    1. frontal         3. parietal
    2. occipital       4. mandible           A B C D E

88. At points where flat bones of the skull meet, there are

    1. cartilaginous joints   3. primary centers
    2. sutures                4. fontanelles   A B C D E

89. Mental retardation may result from

    1. metabolic disturbances     3. fetal infections
    2. chromosomal abnormalities  4. irradiation   A B C D E

# FIVE-CHOICE ASSOCIATION QUESTIONS

DIRECTIONS: Each group of questions below consists of a numbered list of descriptive words or phrases accompanied by a diagram with certain parts indicated by letters, or by a list of lettered headings. For each numbered word or phrase, SELECT THE LETTERED PART OR HEADING that matches it correctly. Then insert the letter in the space to the right of the appropriate number. Sometimes more than one numbered word or phrase may be correctly matched to the same lettered part or heading.

A. Allantois
B. Primitive streak
C. Notochord
D. Blood island
E. Neural plate

90. _____ Gives rise to the brain and spinal cord
91. _____ Source of mesenchyme
92. _____ Rudimentary structure
93. _____ Appears in the wall of the yolk sac

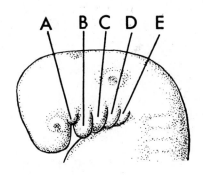

94. _____ Its muscle element gives rise to the muscles of facial expression
95. _____ Its cartilage forms a greater cornu of the hyoid bone
96. _____ Its cartilage gives rise to the styloid process
97. _____ forms the inferior part of the face
98. _____ Gives rise to the lateral palatine process
99. _____ Supplied by the vagus nerve

A. Valve of the foramen ovale
B. Partitions primitive atrium
C. Crista dividens
D. Foramen ovale
E. Umbilical vein

100. _____ Its inferior edge directs blood to the left atrium
101. _____ Carries well oxygenated blood to the fetus
102. _____ Remains of the septum primum
103. _____ Opening in the septum secundum
104. _____ Early septum primum
105. _____ Part of the septum secundum

ASSOCIATION QUESTIONS

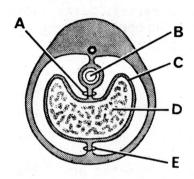

A. Scaphocephaly
B. Apical ectodermal ridge
C. Somatic mesoderm
D. Meromelia
E. Hemivertebra

106. ___ Its free border contains the umbilical vein
107. ___ Embryonic site of hemopoiesis
108. ___ Derived from the foregut and midgut
109. ___ Hepatoduodenal ligament

110. ___ Exerts an inductive influence during limb development
111. ___ Craniosynostosis
112. ___ Partial absence of a limb
113. ___ Limb muscles
114. ___ Scoliosis
115. ___ Premature closure of sagittal suture

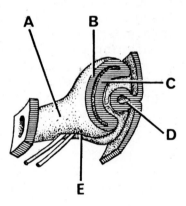

A. Neural crest
B. Alar plates
C. Basal plates
D. Neuroepithelium
E. Spinal ganglion cells

116. ___ Gives rise to the lens
117. ___ Future optic nerve
118. ___ Differentiates into nonpigmented portion of the ciliary epithelium
119. ___ Becomes pigmented layer of the retina
120. ___ Optic fissure
121. ___ Becomes specialized for sensitivity to light

122. ___ Gracile nuclei
123. ___ Form ventral gray columns
124. ___ Neuroglia
125. ___ Unipolar afferent neurons

KEY TO CORRECT RESPONSES

Review Examination

| | | | | | | |
|---|---|---|---|---|---|---|
| 1. B | 19. C | 37. E | 55. C | 73. B | 91. B | 109. A |
| 2. E | 20. A | 38. E | 56. D | 74. E | 92. A | 110. B |
| 3. D | 21. E | 39. C | 57. E | 75. A | 93. D | 111. A |
| 4. B | 22. D | 40. D | 58. A | 76. D | 94. C | 112. D |
| 5. E | 23. C | 41. B | 59. E | 77. C | 95. D | 113. C |
| 6. C | 24. B | 42. E | 60. E | 78. E | 96. C | 114. E |
| 7. A | 25. B | 43. E | 61. B | 79. D | 97. B | 115. A |
| 8. B | 26. D | 44. C | 62. A | 80. C | 98. A | 116. D |
| 9. C | 27. B | 45. A | 63. C | 81. E | 99. E | 117. A |
| 10. E | 28. C | 46. A | 64. A | 82. D | 100. C | 118. C |
| 11. A | 29. A | 47. E | 65. A | 83. A | 101. E | 119. B |
| 12. E | 30. A | 48. A | 66. C | 84. A | 102. A | 120. E |
| 13. C | 31. E | 49. C | 67. E | 85. C | 103. D | 121. C |
| 14. B | 32. D | 50. E | 68. C | 86. D | 104. B | 122. B |
| 15. A | 33. B | 51. C | 69. A | 87. A | 105. C | 123. C |
| 16. D | 34. C | 52. B | 70. E | 88. C | 106. E | 124. D |
| 17. D | 35. E | 53. C | 71. E | 89. E | 107. D | 125. E |
| 18. B | 36. D | 54. A | 72. A | 90. E | 108. B | |

## INTERPRETATION OF YOUR SCORE

| Number of Correct Responses | Level of Performance |
|---|---|
| 107-125 | Excellent - Exceptional |
| 94-106 | Superior - Very Superior |
| 80-93 | Average - Above Average |
| 70-79 | Poor - Marginal |
| 69 or less | Very Poor - Failure |

NOTES

NOTES

NOTES

NOTES

NOTES